WHY
BREATHE

First published in the UK by Breath and Ice Publications 2023
Bristol, UK

Copyright: Gus Hoyt

Gus Hoyt asserts the moral rights to be identified as the author
and illustrator of this work.

A catalogue record of this book is available from the British
Library

ISBN: 978-1-7395314-0-9

Printed and bound in the UK by KDP

WHY

BREATHE

A fun and scientific journey to healthier everyday breathing.
Unlock more energy, reduce stress and live a fuller life

GUS HOYT

Gus Hoyt

Instagram:
@breathandice

With great thanks to everyone who contributed along the way, the list is too long to mention everyone but especial thanks to my wild-swimming buddy Harry who's ear I have talked-off and who read through my first draft and to Sarah who acted as an editor at large. Huge thanks also to Paul who walked me through the self-publishing maze and Joanne who got me over the line.

Thank you to my wonderful and patient editors Ellie Stevenson, Book Coach & Author and Ruth Jewell, Editor and my wonderful cover designer Catherine Clarke, we got there!

Especial thanks to everyone who I have worked with over the years, especially everyone in 'The Tribe of 2020' and all those who continue to question, investigate, share and impart their knowledge onto others and who continue to spread the health and wealth we hold in our breath to the wider community.

Thank you also to the Island of Portland for giving me the space I needed to finish the writing and illustrations.

CONTENTS

"Be curious, not judgemental."

Walt Whitman
(Later, Ted Lasso playing darts)

Introduction

Why am I writing a book? The question we ask ourselves as we stare at the blank pages in front of us, distracted by the birds jumping around outside the window. For me, discovering my breath and the simple tweaks I could incorporate, to unlock the inherent power and possibilities it held, was so transformatory that I have made it a mission to share this with as many people as possible.

There are plenty of excellent and specialist books out there on breathing and breathwork but what I found was that there was nothing there which completely 'spoke' to me. I'm not a yogic, and though I like sports, I am no professional athlete. While working-on and improving my health through my breath, there was a looming gap just aching to be filled - the breathing book for the regular person.

As stressful as the idea of writing (or finishing) a book might seem, this is nothing from what I have experienced at other stages of my life. Now, thanks to realising why we breathe and how to control my nervous system through simple practices, I am now in a position of strength to deal with any challenges and calamity life may throw at me.

So, bring it on, and if you are reading this book you will know that I won that personal battle!

People would see me as a quiet and chilled-out guy but, as is often the case, underneath the surface I was boiling and bubbling away, a constant mire of stress and anxiety. This was my 'normal 'and to match this, as time wore on, I found I needed bigger and stronger activities to stimulate and inspire me. This constant yearning for more drove me into dangerous and destructive territories.

As a child, creativity was my outlet. I could lose myself in the details of a painting or in writing a song. Hours would simply glide by. I could find solace and calm in perfection and order in the fictitious worlds I was creating, but life progresses and responsibilities start to creep-in and then suddenly pile-on. Without realising it, years have gone by and any time for creative output was lost. When time is snatched back we're often too tired to find the flow that once came naturally.

By fault or design my need to chase the next big thing - the next big high - led me into the world of professional kitchens. I worked my way around the world in a life of constant highs and stress, zero hours contracts were the norm, and we were expected to pick-up shifts at the drop of a hat. Or, if the boss was having a bad day, leave and never come back. It was relentless, breakfast was eaten on the go while run-walking to work, or nibbled in between prep and service. This was six or seven days a week and the only holidays we got were when we were fired or quit. We were constantly ON.

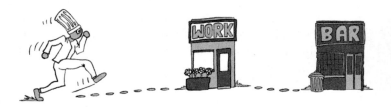

I was chasing the adrenaline rush and over the years this became all I knew. Chasing the high became a learnt behaviour, which stayed with me throughout my life and the many careers I fell into.

From nudging into food campaigning, into the wider field of environmentalism and eventually Green politics and then co-creating a world renowned anti-plastics campaign, I kept this pressure on myself. The need for perfection - and perfection NOW - was the horse leading my chariot.

How to come down again? When you spend 10 hours with your face pressed to a burning grill with orders stacking-up and everyone needing everything *now*, how do you come down from that?! Well, the simple answer would be that you collapse into bed every night - and perhaps that would have been the sensible thing to do.

As chefs, we worked while others had their fun. When we finished - the last order delivered, the grill scrubbed and floors cleaned - the gloves were off... You go out to have *as much fun as you can as quickly as you can* before the bars finally close. Often staying out later still as you're invited to party with the bar staff and local entertainment dancers, who have just finished their shift. Unlike these new friends though, you need to be back at work by 8 or 9am again the next day.

We learn best through repetition. This meant that my learned response to high stress, from my late teens onwards, was to drink copious amounts of booze as fast as I could. The justification was clear and unarguable - to keep that rush going, pushing that pretence at happiness and bringing on the eventual silence and peace of passing-out into a deep sleep. This logic was unarguable but fundamentally flawed and simply wrong.

But we can't stay UP the whole time. While others tried harder, using cocaine to get that extra buzz and keep on going, I just chipped-away on caffeine and pure grit alone. Eventually though, we all hit the same wall. We deplete all our natural stores of adrenalin on a regular basis and we collapse.

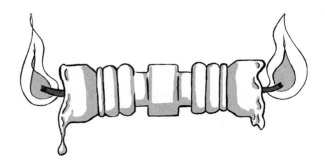

The Zen of 'Work Hard Play Hard'

How very wrong I was. I went from punishing my body at work to punishing it even more after-hours, all in the name of 'balance'.

I burnt the candle at both ends. I threw it into the goddam flames! Then, one day in my mid 30s my alarm went off and yet again I hadn't slept at all. I was sore all over, my head throbbed, my eyes blood-shot and glassy, cheeks swollen and my guts and throat were burning from years of constant acid reflux... and I had to be at work again, to face it all over again for another 10 hours, in under 45 minutes.

Stress and my lifestyle were killing me and I needed to take back control! Things had to change!

Catching my Breath

I fully committed to a program of improvement I devised, an exploratory self-fix programme that came a great deal of introspection, stargazing and trying new practices. One of these was BREATHING.

I realised that the happiest I'd ever been within and of myself, was when I was free and scuba diving down in Dorset. Living in a busy city, with polluted waterways, I couldn't return to this past time, but I could incorporate some of those elements into my daily life. Two of these components: Getting into cold water again and slowing my breathing and doing breath-holds once more were to change my life beyond recognition!

This started a journey down a rabbit-hole into the many facets of breathing and breathwork and many other related activities. While deep down there I rediscovered - almost like a eureka moment - WHY we actually breathe in the first place, how and why we're getting it wrong and therefore what we can do about it to change things around.

Along the way I made lots of blunders. I bought lots of expensive gizmos ranging from sports masks that made me look like a Batman villain to apps that listened to me sleep. These did nothing but distract me from the simple act of breathing itself, but in the end the truth that comes with finding my breath was returned to me and I haven't looked back.

These are the things I'm going to share here in this book: simple explanations, easy exercises and roads to recovery and a way to help you better understand your breath, and therefore harnessing the immense power you have over your life. I'll skip the jargon and technical terminology, avoid over-complicating terminology and will get straight to the point.

Rarely is the answer directly under our nose.

Through accessing my breath I have found my balance. My mind has calmed and I can *feel* the homeostasis (the literal balance of bodily systems) within my body. Balance I may have found, but this isn't some zen master sitting under a tree kinda stuff. This is everyday breathing and breathwork exercises, which we can do anywhere from sitting on a bus to watching TV. I'll share all that has brought me balance - or, as I like to call it, a state of readiness - an ability to meet the world head on and be able to bring myself up, down or straight ahead depending on my needs at the time. I am back in control of my body and mind - they are no longer spiralling out of control!

Hiding from Nature

An important thing to mention, and I'll come back to this a few times, is that we are animals. We like to dress things up (ourselves included) and pretend we are above the rest of the animal world, that we are on an elevated platform, but we aren't. We are animals. We have exactly the same functions as every other mammal that walks the earth and we have the same basic responses to danger as they do too.

The difference is that we have created for ourselves thousands of stressors throughout the day, that tap into and trigger this ancient danger response. By artificially living in cities and larger than normal communities, through our invention and use of money, technology and an expanding intellect, we became our own worst enemies and it's slowly killing us and the planet we live on.

Our bodies interpret these 'micro-stressors 'as danger and this prompts the natural stress response to kick-in. In today's world this has led to anxiety, illness, mental health problems and even early death. We are not in danger when an email pops-up from our boss, but that's how our animal self interprets it, and this is where a lot of the problems begin - but more on that later.

We consistently interpret so many things as threats. Our nervous system is in a constantly elevated state of arousal - or stress - and this has a plethora of damaging consequences. We don't need to be a chef or an NHS nurse to feel these stressors, they are all around us in our daily lives.

Through my personal exploration of this topic, and talking to the people I have met as clients and guests in my workshops, it is clear that this problem is at pandemic proportions and yet so few of us are looking at, let alone addressing the core root of our problems.

We are animals but we are no longer behaving or breathing like them, and this leads to problems.

From feeling unpleasant and unproductive all day at work, to developing illness, addictions, fatigue, mental health problems and early death - poor breathing is at the core of it all. We look at our diet, we exercise more, we rub lotions into our skin and we rely on robotic instruments to monitor our lives, but something we consistently overlook is that simple thing we do over 20,000 times a day!

In the medical profession, everyone is aware of breathing disorders when they become severe, or ill health itself affects our breathing. But only more recently, starting with the Ukrainian physiologist Buteyko in the 1950s, has it been noted that this is a 'positive (or negative) feedback loop 'and what that means is that bad or poor breathing in itself can start us on the road to illness.

Breathing is not something to be sniffed at - and again: the answer lies right in front of us.

Our modern lifestyle has led to inappropriate, inefficient and dangerous breathing patterns, affecting our diet, lifestyle and the way we live. They have spiralled out of our control and we haven't even noticed. Our maladies may be as simple as a feeling of fog or lack of concentration and focus, but they can manifest into much more serious conditions if left unchecked.

However, we have the power to change this. Bad habits that take decades to create can be undone and even reversed surprisingly quickly. These same feedback loops that plunge us into poor health, can quickly be turned on their head, and we can install healthy and nurturing practices where previously damaging ones thrived.

Chapter 1
Why/How do we Breathe
in the First Place?

You may be thinking why the hell do you need to read a book on breathing? You wouldn't be alone, while talking with friends and strangers alike, when I say I'm a Breathwork Coach the person I'm with will often puff-out a few pantomime breaths, laugh and say something like:

'And how's that working out for you? I've been breathing all my life and I'm not dead yet!'

And this is true - but should 'I'm not dead yet' *really* be the benchmark that we strive towards - or should we maybe be aiming a little higher?

They are correct though. We all breathe over 20,000 times a day without a second thought. So, why *are* we talking about breathing?

Breathing is something we just do without having to think about it. It's often something we pay very little notice to until it's too late. Until we 'lose 'our breath or breathing becomes difficult through injury, fatigue or illness, we don't pay the blindest bit of notice to this activity. We just do it without having to think about it. Classically, we don't know what we've got untill it's gone, but why not stop it from doing us harm, why not maximise it while we still have it, *before* it is too late?

Unlike our diet, breathing is not something we focus on. We've been bombarded our whole lives to think about what we eat, what we put in our body through our mouths. It's a multi-billion dollar industry with millions of vested interests. Just as every bite of food we take can be 'good 'or 'bad 'for us, every breath can be positive or negative for our health. As we take so many breaths a day, maybe it's time we started thinking about it a little more.

It's worth noting that not *every* bite of food and every breath is going to kill us, or lead us to salvation. An extra glass of wine with friends or a chocolate bar when we're feeling lonely isn't going to tip the scales! It can be unhealthy to think like that, but the cumulative effects over days, weeks, years and decades does.

Just by reading this or any book on breathing, you've already taken a massive first step forward. This positive change in thinking will guide us slowly towards greater awareness, understanding and overall health. From this point on, whatever your previous thoughts on the subject, you'll notice and think about your breath a whole lot more - and that's an excellent first step!

So let's look at the basics first. We can't build a house unless it has good foundations, so let's start at the ground and build our way up.

In my workshops my favourite question to ask is simply "Why do we breathe?"

So, close your eyes, put down the book and think to yourself for a moment, why DO we breathe - and there are no wrong answers at this point.

When we ask ourselves "Why do we breathe?" most of us say:" To bring air in and out of the body", "to breathe in air/oxygen" or "to bring oxygen into the body and get rid of excess carbon dioxide" - or something along those lines. You may also have said:" To give us energy" or "so we can live/so we don't die." All of these are correct and, for now, bang on the mark!

One simple definition of WHY we breathe could be: To bring increased levels of oxygen (O_2) into our lungs. This oxygen passes into our blood, which is then pumped by our heart around our body. In exchange for the oxygen, carbon dioxide (CO_2) as a waste product ,is then carried away from the cells in our blood back via our heart to our lungs, which we then exhale - or breathe out.

This is the most basic answer to our question and is more of a 'How we breathe'. As such, we'll come back and expand on some of this later on, but does it really answer the question as to WHY we breathe?

My apologies if this is triggering to parents of toddlers who are constantly bombarded with 'Why?" questions but this is important. The above is what happens when we breathe but WHY do we breathe?

We breathe to supply oxygen to our cells, so that they can convert it with glucose into energy. Without oxygen we couldn't create energy in our cells. Without being able to create energy in our cells they would wither and die. ***We*** *would wither and die.*

This is the most basic answer as to why we breathe. Does this mean we can pop this book back on the shelf now? As you can possibly guess by the page number, there's still plenty more for us to look at.

As with most answers of course, this just raises more questions, starting with how does this work and why is breathing so important in making energy and keeping us alive?

Creating Energy

Every cell in our body includes a little 'factory 'in it called mitochondria. These are the power houses that generate life itself - or enable it to happen, almost everything that happens in the human body gets its energy from here. When we breathe, the oxygen is carried around our body in the bloodstream and it 'delivers 'this oxygen to where it is needed or where it's in demand. From here it is delivered to the mitochondria and turned into energy.

But nothing happens in isolation in our bodies. At the same time, glucose is extracted from the food we eat and is absorbed into the blood. Like the oxygen, it is distributed to our cells and delivered to our mitochondria. This is where the 'magic ' happens. The mitochondria takes the oxygen and the glucose and through chemical processes, creates energy out of it.

Glucose + Oxygen = Energy with the by-products of Carbon Dioxide and Water.

For the more science minded, the exact equation is opposite:

$$C6H12O6 + 6O2 = ATP \text{ (ENERGY) and } 6CO2 + 6H2O$$

We deliver oxygen to our cells, it combines with glucose and this creates usable energy (or Adenosine triphosphate/ATP) which is the condensed energy for cells to use. During this process, there are the by-products of carbon dioxide, which we then breathe out and water, which is both exhaled and simply absorbed back into our blood and body.

Now we have a basic and most essential 'WHY?', let's move deeper into the 'HOW? 'and see where this journey takes us.

An Internal Ballet

So, we breathe in to supply our cells with energy. This sounds simple but like all things simple in life, it is actually incredibly complex. This connection of processes and interconnected systems and body parts work together in a ballet that is worthy of the Royal Opera House. This is a process that goes on twenty four hours a day, seven days a week and happens for the most part entirely unseen (talk about the hidden stars of the show!).

A healthy body will always try and find a state of equilibrium - or homeostasis. Our mind continually tries to confuse things but, our body will always seek this balance. One really interesting example of this is in our blood. We'll only have time to have a little look into this beautiful interplay here.

We breathe in, oxygen-rich air comes into our lungs, making its way down the ever-decreasing branches to tiny little pockets or air sacs known as alveoli (not to be confused with the delicious garlic condiment 'aioli'). Here, the oxygen passes through a permeable membrane into the blood vessels that circulate around them. At the same time carbon dioxide switches place with the oxygen from the blood and is then able to be breathed out.

Simple right? Great. So let's follow that oxygen now it's in our blood and see where it goes, how it travels and how it knows where it needs to be delivered in the body.

Before we do this let's look at our blood. Our blood is made-up of many components, but we want to look at is the most common aspect of blood, our red blood cells (RBCs). They are concave disks - similar to an American donut but with a thin layer connecting the hole in the middle. Right, we're all thinking about donuts now... but... red blood cells...

These cells contain haemoglobin, which is a protein bond that connects with the chemicals of our breath. It bonds onto the oxygen molecules and holds them in place. I like to think of haemoglobin as seats on the bus, which is a red blood cell. A lovely blood-coloured bus.

There needs to be a space for the oxygen to bond with the red blood cells. There needs to be free seats on the bus, for the oxygen to get on board. These molecules are *really* eager to get on the bus, so when there's space, where there's a seat, they're there!

Ding-ding. Let's go!

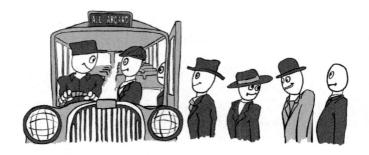

Like a bus taking on passengers, the red blood cells carry oxygen and carbon dioxide where they need to go in the body

And off we set. The oxygen happily bobbing along on the bus, singing a song and merrily going along its way. The oxygen is so happy on the bus that it will keep on riding until it's time to get off. But, like a tourist in a new city it needs help to know where to get off. Where is its stop?
This is where one of the very clever interplays comes into action.

Remember that Oxygen + Glucose = Energy + Carbon Dioxide?

This means that once energy has been created in the cell, once the supply of oxygen has been used-up, it will give off carbon dioxide. Suddenly the thumb is out and the carbon dioxide is standing impatiently at the bus stop waiting to go home (back to the lungs and out into the air to be inhaled by a tree, or a blob of algae). The molecule is tired, it's done its work and it *really* wants to go home.

When the bus, or red blood cells ladened with oxygen, comes along it aggressively forces its way on board. In doing so, as the carbon dioxide boards it forces the oxygen molecule off. Carbon dioxide is able to break the bond that oxygen has with the haemoglobin. This means that when and where there is an excess of carbon dioxide, if oxygen rich blood comes along, they will switch places before the bus trundles all the way back to the lungs.

And that's it. We inhale the oxygen, it bonds to the blood, and is carried to the parts of the body that are active and using oxygen to create energy based on need. Then the carbon dioxide that is the byproduct of energy production breaks the bond, jumps on the bus and the fresh oxygen finds its stop and joins in the party.
And so on. This beautiful ballet continues and would put to shame any city's public transport system. And it all goes on beneath our skin without us even noticing. Brilliant!

(Now, of course it can get a little bit more complicated, but we'll come back to that later.)

Chapter 2
What *is* a Deep Breath?

Where it All Begins

As a sickly kid I was often in my doctors surgery. Most sessions would start with me standing there, shirtless and waiting for him to place an ice-cold stethoscope on my chest before asking me to 'Take a nice deep breath'.

I would inhale as dramatically as I could. Puffing out my chest, drawing up my shoulders and arching my back as I sucked that air deeply in.

He would lazily nod as he gazed off into the distance and listened to whatever strange and mysterious noises were coming to his ears through the stethoscope.

He was my GP. I fully trusted him and would smile to myself that I had done a good job. I'd been a good boy.

Just like that, this became my benchmark for 'a nice deep breath'. This remained unchanged for many decades until I was much older and a luckily a lot wiser.

Looking back I cannot fathom why my doctor would have encouraged such reckless abandon around my taking of a deep breath, and the health implications it was to have on my life. But hindsight is a powerful lens, and with consideration I realise it wasn't his fault. Back when he became a doctor, few people trained in breathwork or studied the holistic medicines or therapies, which are more prevalent and mainstream now.

He was probably just thinking about getting another of these assessments done, so he could go to the pub for a ploughman's or go and eat his sandwiches in a nearby field... but this could also just be my rose-tinted lenses of the 'good old days 'as propagated by the Ladybird books we were force-fed as children. Either way, he wasn't 100% present during these assessments.

Luckily now, our knowledge has improved and we understand things a bit better. In today's world, this would be a very dangerous pattern for any health care professional to encourage.

Most of us will take our doctor's advice as gospel (unless it's cutting back on drinking and fun foods) and especially so at an early age. It's essential that more training, support and funding is given to our NHS, so that we can continue to build on the amazing thing they created 75 years ago.

Deep = Furthest from the Surface

A deep breath is filling-up our lungs, starting from the lowest point possible and working our way upwards from there.

In physiological terms, this would mean taking a breath in as high as possible into the lowest point of the lungs imaginable. So: In through the nose and deep down into the bottom part of your lungs.

As a diver, the easiest way for me to understand a deep breath is to think of the ocean. What is the deepest part? Quite simply it is the point at which the distance between the top and the bottom, the surface and the floor, the waves and the seabed, are at their greatest.

Or put more simply: 'Deep is far from the surface'.

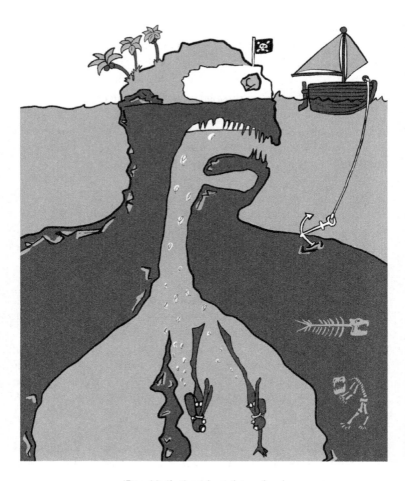

'Deep' is 'furthest from the surface'

In physiological terms, this would mean taking a breath in as high as possible into the lowest point of the lungs imaginable. So: In through the nose and deep down into the bottom part of your lungs. It really is as simple as that!

Follow your Nose

We'll cover both the nose and the diaphragm in separate chapters, but as for this amazing thing in the middle of your face, let's have a quick look at *why and how* breathing through the nose makes it specifically a deep breath.

As we inhale through our nose the air is warmed, moistened and filtered ready to go into our body proper. It is directed in and up through a structure of turbines (or 'turbulates') that prepare the flow, so that when it hits our throat it is travelling smoothly and gently straight down. Compare this with a mouth breath that directs the air straight back into our throat, and causes minor trauma to both the larynx and trachea as it hits them, and we can already see what a good job nasal breathing is doing.

So the air is taken in, up further into our nasal cavity, prepared for our lungs and then it is effortlessly and safely transported deep down to our lungs with the use of a nice diaphragmatic 'belly breath'.

Lung Shape and Space Available

Let's now take a quick but comprehensive look at our lungs. Our respiratory system is basically made out of breathing tubes, that split and divide as they descend from head to alveoli. Our breath ideally starts in our nose but possibly in our mouth, and it descends down through our trachea (a dead-space of around 150ml) and then divides into our main left and right bronchus. From here they continue to branch-off into different smaller and narrower tubes or bronchi until they get to the smallest denominator, the bronchioles, which are between 0.5 and 5mm thick.

The lungs can look like upside-down and slightly wonky trees. The trunk starts large and keeps dividing all the way down, till it gets to the leaves at the end of the branches and twigs/bronchioles and alveoli. This shouldn't be the magical and mystical revelation that it so often is. Trees evolved in the same world as our lungs. We aren't separate from nature but are a part of it, and so we have evolved the way we have.

Just like trees have leaves, we have little air sacs called alveoli and these amazing organs have a combined surface area of a football pitch - all cleverly scrunched-up inside our two little lungs. The walls of our alveoli are semi permeable membranes, which allow the passing of gases, most importantly oxygen and carbon dioxide, to enter into our bloodstream via capillaries and veins that encompass them.

If we imagine that healthy tree, growing up towards the sun and sky and flip it upside-down, we can see that the part of the lungs with the greatest surface area - and therefore the most efficient part of the lungs for us to inhale into, is the bottom third. This is where the most alveoli are located and also where we find the majority of blood capillaries. Their thin walls, semi-permeable membranes are able to seamlessly transfer the oxygen and carbon dioxide from the air in our lungs to the blood in our 'veins'. It's so perfect in design, it is almost as if we were designed by a brilliant scientist in a lab somewhere.

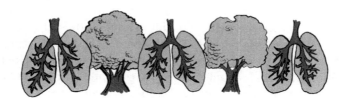

Working in Harmony

Quite simply put, a deep breath is when we breathe into our nose and down into the bottom part/third of our lungs. As we breathe through the nose the airflow is slowed down, it takes time to get all the way down into the bottom of our lungs as they slowly inflate. This allows for oxygen to be properly delivered via the membranes into our blood and for the carbon dioxide to hitch a ride back out again. We lose less volume of each breath due to the dead-space in our throats, so that even though we breathe less times than if we were breathing fast into our chest, we are getting more air delivered to the parts that matter.

Let's think of that bus analogy again. The blood flowing around our body carrying oxygen and carbon dioxide where it needs to go - where we need it most. If the bus flies into the station at 100mph before doing a handbrake skid, we aren't going to see many passengers able to get safely off and on. Many will be stuck where they are and if they do get off they will be so shaken by the experience that this feeling of panic will stay with them, and get communicated throughout the rest of the passengers, until we have a full blown freak-out on a speeding bus. But this time Keanu isn't at the wheel.

This is a nice atmospherically-controlled bus, pulling up carefully and slowly into the station to calmly let passengers off, with plenty of time for the new ones to get on, sit down comfortably and make sure they have all of their luggage.

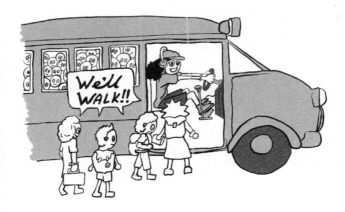

EXERCISE

Let's see how that feels for ourselves. See if you can just breathe in and out through your nose. If you can't, no worries, just slow your breath down a little. Let's close our eyes and imagine all those red blood cell buses zooming round our body.

Like with a remote control car, we have the button in our hands, let's ease-off on the power, breathing lighter, softer, allowing all those oxygen molecules to get safely on and off again.
Can you feel the difference?

All combined, this simple 'deep breath 'allows for maximum gas exchange with minimum energy expended. So a deep breath is also a slower breath, it's an efficient breath. It is an effective and trauma-free breath and one that gives us maximum benefit for minimum effort.

A true deep breath, also brings with it a whole plethora of related and unrelated benefits but we'll dive into these soon enough. If our body is 'designed 'to take natural deep breaths, and it's easier and healthier for us to do so, what exactly is standing in our way? Why do we even need to talk about it in the first place - let alone as a public health necessity?

Negative Cultural Influences/Does my Breath Look Fat in This?

In our culture we are told to puff out our chest, push back our shoulders and suck in our belly. I say in our culture - to clarify: I am a white anglo-American who was born in the late '70s. But this is viewed pretty universally.

Whether male or female, we are encouraged to push out our chest and pull in our belly, and people from many different cultures I have spoken to attest that this was the same for them - so it goes beyond my small personal cultural experience.

We all have an aversion to looking fat. We spend far too much time and money on worrying about, and trying to fix, this perceived problem and this is taking its toll on our healthy breathing patterns. Whether it is fad diets, supplements instead of foods, buying expensive watches that tell us to walk more or surgery and more invasive methods and technologies. We are, it is safe to say, somewhat obsessed.

Now, don't get me wrong, there are a LOT of health problems associated with chronic obesity, including increased pressure on our respiratory and cardio-vascular systems, but I'm talking about our obsession with 'feeling fat 'when there is little or no problem at all. We are supposed to have insulation around us and fat is also our energy storage for the lean times. It is just that our culture, or the advertising industry and the fear they prey on, that has steered us towards both overeating and making unhealthy food choices, then immediately being consumed by guilt and self-loathing. But this isn't a diet book.

We are overly obsessed by body image and overpowered with a paranoid feeling that we are 'too fat'. We are constantly and consistently bombarded with advertising, magazine articles, social media posts, tv shows and big screen movies - all of them populated with almost cartoon-proportioned heroes and leading stars. All perfect teeth and zero body fat.

This constant onslaught has affected almost every part of our life, even including our healthy breathing patterns. Ironically, as we'll explore later, inefficient breathing will lead to poor digestion and sugar cravings, however that's not what we're talking about here.

'Are you beach-body ready?' Influencers and models sucking in their gut dangerously, during seemingly 'natural 'poses has normalised this very abnormal body image we all now hold for ourselves in the mirror.

What we *are* talking about here, is body image directly affecting the mechanics of our breath and the problems this can create for a healthy and functional breathing pattern. We have three levels of breathing muscles, helpfully labelled primary, secondary and tertiary. Social pressures are forcing us to turn this scale upside down and it is having terrible consequences on our daily health.

Our primary breathing muscles are our diaphragm - an incredible breathing muscle connected at the base of our lungs. As it contracts, it draws down and increases the volume in the chest capacity, creating a vacuum and this in turn draws air into the lungs.

In partnership with our diaphragm are our intercostal muscles. These serve to further open our lungs, drawing more air in. There are muscles both on the outside and inside of our ribs, sitting between the bones themselves (think about the meaty bits on a BBQ plate of spare-ribs). When these external muscles contract they pull outwards, this expands the volume of our chest capacity and draws more air in, conversely, if we need to forcibly exhale, the internal muscles will contract.

Though we *can* forcibly exhale by contracting the diaphragm the other way, and using the muscles on the inside of our ribs, there's not much call for it. In most everyday breathing, a simple relaxation after the inhale allows us to return to a neutral position, ready for the next breath.

These primary breathing muscles expand the bottom part of our lungs which, as we know, are the richest and most efficient part to breathe into. This is the most efficient and effective breath we can take. It is a relaxed and text-book 'deep breath'.

Then there are the secondary breathing muscles: these support the primary muscles in their task, and ideally, if unobstructed, lead to a fuller breath. This group includes the pectorals and

intercostals in our upper chest and our larger back muscles.
Lastly, and only in times of extreme need, there are the tertiary breathing muscles which are in our clavicles, neck, shoulders and upper-upper chest. These only kick in when we are absolutely gasping for breath - remember the last time you had to *really* sprint and were left bent double and gasping for air - with a feeling of exhaustion, light-headedness and/or stress and fear? That's the gasping breath and it's only ever naturally employed when we really really need it.

It gets the essential job done but breathing like this isn't sustainable and is dangerous in the long term.

As Patrick McKeown says: *'If your shoulders move while you're breathing, that's a clear sign of dysfunctional breathing.'*

Sadly though, in our culture we *are* constantly told to suck in our belly. This means not using our diaphragm to breathe or not using it properly. Whether male or female we're told to push out our chest as this is a sign of attractiveness. Instead of a nurturing belly breath, this leads to us breathing into our chest, as it is a lot easier than several months worth of press-ups and cheaper than surgery (though a padded bra is maybe a healthier option). It's so ingrained that even after these exercises and procedures, influencers still maintain this 'suck n puff' pose.

Coupled with all these pressures is the design of our clothes themselves. When our clothes are skin tight, it can just exacerbates the problem we already have with how we look when we breathe. The overly tight clothing may also restricts the movement of a healthy breath.

We can also develop problems due to restrictions caused by the belts we wear, restrictive trouser waistlines, braces ('suspenders' for my American friends - something very different for English speakers) and worst of all - corsets! (As much of a fan as I am of Dita Von Teese, there's a reason women were regularly passing-out in the Victorian Age, though many may have also used it as a ploy to avoid toxic men.)

This means we are essentially breathing upside-down, we're breathing back to front. We are prioritising the least effective and least efficient breathing muscles, over muscles that will never tire. This is known as 'Paradoxical Breathing 'and it is a form of dysfunctional breathing and one that is rife today.

Breathing is the New Black

There's good news though! It certainly isn't all doom and gloom. Paradoxical Breathing is easy to fix. It's relatively simple to undo years or even decades of bad breathing, just by flipping this on its head and learning how to breathe again properly, naturally and effectively. Like everything in life, the more we practise, the better we will become and before we know it, we are doing it subconsciously and naturally.

We'll soon look at how Breathing, the Nervous System, and the Stress Response affect one another in the body. We'll also look at how paradoxical breathing plays a very negative role here, driving-up our stress levels, and creating a society that is more on edge and prone to burn out and collapse - something I can attest to personally, but for now let's just look at how inefficient this is.

We have evolved to breathe into the lower part of our lungs. This is where the majority of the alveoli are, this is where the majority of the blood capillaries are and this is where the strongest and least tiring muscles are located. We'd be hard pressed to say that we could design a better system if we tried. This is where the roads are clearer, the most buses can get through and there are plenty of nice relaxed bus stops for our red blood cells to use.

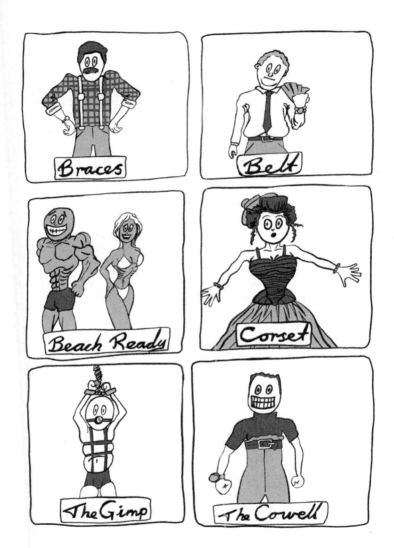

The clothes we wear can restrict our natural breath

Breathing into the chest and shoulders however, is the least effective way to draw air into our body. It uses loads more energy and is the least efficient way to breathe. From an evolutionary perspective alone this should be reason enough to move away from this foolish obsession - but as we'll learn later it is also slowly killing us and driving us towards chronic illness and sub-optimal living.

Now we're aware of it, it is super simple to reverse. We just need to give ourselves space to breathe and permission to let our bellies expand that little bit more when we inhale. Forget the influencers with zero body fat telling us to suck it in! Let it go, enjoy your breath! A healthy breath IS a path to freedom and health, mood and life itself. So let that belly swell beautifully with every breath.

As every beautiful, confident and healthy breath begins with our diaphragm, perhaps it's time for us to have a closer look at this wonderful and oft overlooked muscle.

Chapter 3
The Diaphragm

I 'Heart 'Diaphragm

As we breathe in using our diaphragm it contracts and pulls down. The vital role it plays here, as we discussed, is to create a vacuum above and draw air in. However, it also performs many other wonderful functions and that's why we all need to fall a bit more in love with the diaphragm.

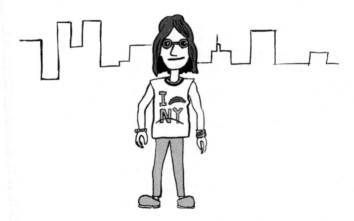

Our heart is amazing and of course we need to care for and love it, but maybe we should all be wearing t-shirts with a diaphragm on it instead of a heart. Why? Well, because it is this part of our body that is most responsible for self regulation and love. And, as we all know, we can't really experience true love for others until we learn to love ourselves first - and this must be true as I read it on a tea-towel!

But seriously - our primary breathing muscle does SO much more than just help pull air into our body.

As we take a nice deep breath - go on, let's take another one together now, close your eyes and breathe nice and deep. What do you notice?

Feel into your body and see what happens. Take a few more nice deep breaths. Really feel into it - OK, now put down the book and try it.

I'm guessing that you felt a few things. First off, a physical sensation of your belly expanding - like a lovely pot-bellied pig. As we inhale, our belly 'grows'. This is why it's kind of mistakenly (or lovingly) called a 'belly breath 'but what actually is at play here?

Where the Breath Begins

If asked: 'Where does your breath begin?' you might answer with your mouth or your nose, but these are just the spaces the air is drawn in through. The breath begins with a friend of ours and it's time for us to get reacquainted with our diaphragm.

The diaphragm is one of those parts of the body that continues to amaze me. As soon as we think we understand it, along comes another function and role that it plays in our general well-being. Considering how important it is, the diaphragm to me is more exciting than our heart - and that's a pretty bold statement to make.

So what is it? In *very* basic terms it's a convex muscle that sits under our lungs. Though it's often said to be an umbrella shape, if we're going to get technical about it, our diaphragm is more like one of those aerodynamic, unbreakable storm umbrellas, and it is one of our most important primary breathing muscles.

Our diaphragm acts as a barrier to separate our upper thoracic cavity (lungs and heart) from our other vital organs, such as our stomach, kidneys, liver and the rest of our 'guts 'in our abdomen. That said there are a number of holes in our diaphragm that allow our major artery, vein and oesophagus to pass through. Unlike an umbrella though, these holes are carefully designed and don't (or shouldn't) allow any leakages. They are tight and secure.

It's a muscle that will never tire - or never get a stitch - and is directly wired-into our Autonomic Nervous System (ANS) and is connected to our heart and brain. As such our diaphragm and its actions affects almost every function in the body. And yet, even when *we are* thinking about it, we often don't really give it much more credit than being a simple breathing muscle - like a bicep for our lungs.

As we understand more about the relationship between the diaphragm and the rest of the body, we can start to see how conscious breathwork and being aware of our breathing can help to shape our health and vitality all across the board. More than a Eureka moment this is like the crescendo of a NYE firework display!

That's some bold talk there, but this humble muscle has the brawn to back it up! Let's dive a little deeper.

As the diaphragm contracts - and for this purpose let's simplify things and think of it in two dimensions - it moves from a convex shape and flattens out. As this happens, it pulls down on the thoracic membrane it is connected to, which increases the volume of the thoracic cavity above and it is this process that draws the air in. (Think of a set of bellows. When they are opened the internal area grows in size/volume and air rushes in.)

If we stop here for a moment, this is the point where we can hear the first of many pennies drop. As the volume increases, the air is sucked into the lungs through the pressure differential that is created. This means that the breath *starts* in the lungs (ideally with the diaphragm) and *not* through the nose or mouth as we often believe - these are 'just the holes 'in which the air can enter the body.

When we take a nice deep healthy breath, we breathe in through our diaphragm.

EXERCISE
So let's try it. Closing our eyes again, let's feel that lovely breathing muscle in our belly. Bringing our awareness into our breath, can you feel the diaphragm as it contracts, pulling our lungs down, expanding them and massaging our guts?

Let's just take a few breaths here, as we focus on our diaphragm.
And smile.

Now obviously there are huge benefits to nasal breathing as we have already started to touch on but, we do not breathe in through the nose, *we breathe in from the diaphragm.* Once we get our heads around this the very idea of our breath is literally turned upside-down. If we have any lingering anxieties around our nose we can relax and start to consciously take control a *lot* more easily.

And just as we breathe in through our diaphragm, we then start to use the rest of our primary breathing muscles - these are our intercostal muscles connected to the inside and outside of our ribs. But the breath should ideally always start with the diaphragm - how many times more can I say diaphragm in this chapter? As many as it takes!

360 Degrees of Breath

A healthy and deep breath starts low and expands upwards and outwards but, not too far. If we consistently employ our secondary or tertiary breathing muscles (around our upper chest, upper back) then we are becoming less efficient and may be starting to edge into a stressful or overstimulated breath or we could risk over-breathing which causes a whole raft of problems in itself.

As soon as our shoulders get involved - and worse still, our neck, then we are well and truly in dysfunctional breathing territory - unless we have just run for our life and are catching our breath, but even still…

So, from a mechanical point of view, a deep breath starts with the diaphragm and then expands upwards and outwards, employing the ribs (external intercostals to be specific) and muscles in the lower back. This is sometimes described as a 'donut breath' as it is similar to a ring donut - however if I was ever served a donut in that shape I'd send it straight back to the kitchen.

As chance or intelligent design (well, evolution) would have it, this is also where the majority of the thin capillaries are situated, which allows for the most efficient location for gaseous exchange to occur. Plainly put, carbon dioxide leaves the body from our blood into our lungs and out again, and oxygen enters our body through the reverse direction - into our nose/mouth, down our trachea and bronchioles and into our lungs, down to the alveoli and then across the permeable membranes into our blood.

So a nice deep diaphragmatic breath allows us to draw in the most air possible, using the least amount of effort/energy and delivering it to the most dense areas of alveoli, thereby giving us the best gas exchange possible.

Best to think of it as a 360 breath - or a nice full inhalation all around the core of our body.

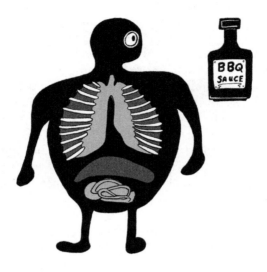

Our diaphragm sits below our lungs and
intercostal muscles in between our ribs

Core and Spine Stabilisation

The benefits of Functional Breathwork don't simply revolve
around the efficiency of our breath - there are plenty of
secondary benefits and knock-on effects. One of these is core
stability. It's pretty much understood and widely cited now but
still worth covering.

When we take a breath in, if we then hold it under pressure this
gives our core a great deal of extra stability and strength. This
is required for many types of physical activities. It provides a
strong base to throw or lift something and for dynamic moves
like rolls and jumps. The deep breath adds support to our spine
and vulnerable lower back muscles.

Early in my gym membership, my personal trainer described it in super-simple and non-technical terms and I've yet to hear a better explanation. Though I was running a campaign to end single-use plastic bottles at the time they were still all over the gym (and sadly still are) and he picked one up to demonstrate his point:

The empty plastic bottle is just a shell and we can think of our lungs in the same way - a thin covering that holds 'nothing but air'. If the bottle is full of air and we take the top off and apply pressure it crumples. It has zero structural integrity. However, if it is full of nothing but air and we keep the lid securely screwed-on it's going to be almost impossible to crush. Its structural strength is greatly increased by a factor of thousands.

The same is true of our lungs and the added support they can give us. If we inhale and hold that breath, then we hold the pressure within. This takes a lot of the load off our muscles and also adds a flexible stability that adds rigidity to our core but doesn't add so much that we might break.

This added stability is seen in its crudest form in the most brutal of moves like deadlifts and squats - inhale in, hold and push/pull, letting out a little air so you don't burst or rupture something as you go. It can also be seen more subtly in the contact sports from boxing to Taekwondo. Those practicing Taekwondo were early adopters of functional breathwork and its benefits on and off the mat. This was mostly because of the mastery and development of techniques championed by Rickson Gracie of Brazilian Jiu-Jitsu fame.

A Belly and Detox Massage

A belly breath does a lot more than just putting a bit of pressure on our belts and creating some funny thoughts about feeling fat, we are also getting a lovely internal massage. All of our 'insides', our vital organs associated with digestion, are below the thoracic membrane. When the diaphragm pulls down it squishes them slightly and helps gently move everything along in the right direction, stopping blockages and keeping things flowing.

Conversely, if we only take shallow chest breaths which is common in our modern sedimentary and office-based lives, then our guts just sit there and sulk.

As we're no longer spending all day walking, foraging, gathering firewood, playing, dancing and maybe (if you're a 'red in tooth and claw 'guy) - hunting, our guts spend a lot of time just sitting there. Sitting has been compared to 'the new smoking 'on so many levels. We were designed to move and living a sedentary life is contrary to our millions of years of evolution.

Without moving naturally, blood flow can become restricted, food travelling through our intestines can get blocked, building-up pressure and also inhibiting the break-down and absorption of nutrients. Waste materials aren't filtered efficiently and slowly build-up in the blood and guts, leading to additional potential problems, but we have an inbuilt tool to help overcome these problems… our diaphragm!

As we inhale deeply we are literally giving our guts a lovely massage.

By giving a nice and regular bit of pressure from above, we are literally giving them a vital, gentle and loving massage. We are applying, then releasing pressure and helping release any knots and kinks just like when a stocky masseur goes to task on our backs and shoulders. Releasing tension and blockages is essential in all parts of the body and none more so than our digestive system.

Our digestive system and tract is under assault from all areas of modern life - from processed food, added sugars, chemicals and artificial additives to meat dependency and lack of fibre etc, but this is a book on breathing so I'll leave you to discover all the wonderful books on nutrition, our gut and microbiome or 'good bacteria' in your next read (see the bibliography and suggested further reading at the end of this book for tips). We just shouldn't add to all these problems with an unnatural breath as well.

The delightful internal massages don't stop here. By employing a nice flowing deep breath starting at the diaphragm we also gently help to drain the toxins and then move the lymphatic fluid along through our body. Unlike our circulatory system, which is driven by the heart, our lymphatic system requires the movement of our body to squeeze the 'waste 'liquid along through tubes with valves to stop back-flow, to our liver and kidneys.

As well as muscular movement, a nice full breath is essential in moving this waste fluid to its end processing plant in the kidneys and liver before being excreted. In many yogic traditions deep diaphragmatic breaths are used as a means of detoxing. By both ensuring a healthy blood and lymphatic flow, we are able to encourage the toxins that build-up in our body and are expelled both through our breath as well as traditional methods of pee and poo.

We are reminded of our body's ability to exhale toxins every time we meet a friend who is worse for wear after a heavy night's drinking, or by his/her health-conscious friend who is on a keto diet. The fumes leaving both their bodies are distinctive and something to avoid direct contact with. Often we can also 'smell 'when friends and colleagues are ill. As we are social animals, this is a clear sensory signal along similar lines to our face going red when we eat something that is poisonous, or that we are allergic to. Breath mint anyone?

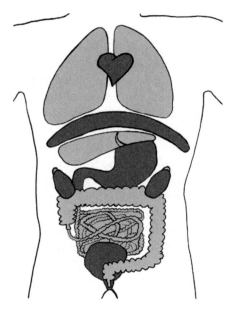

Our internal organs: *lungs, heart,
diaphragm, liver, stomach, kidneys and
adrenal glands, big and small intestines
and bladder*

But feel back into that nice deep breath - go on, close your eyes
again and feel into it. Feel the pressure and release? Feel the
belly growing then relaxing back into place. Feel the movement
in the lower abdomen? Feels great huh?

So, by consciously (or unconsciously) breathing lower into our
bodies we are relying on our most prime or premium breathing
muscles and in doing so we are giving our guts a lovely delicious
and nurturing massage, which is even more important these
days due to our predisposition to sitting in/on chairs.

Vagus Nerve and Relaxation

Something else fun happens when we breathe deeply using our diaphragm: We relax. We'll look into stress in more detail later, as it certainly deserves its own chapter but while we are talking about massaging our guts, let's have a quick look at how else diaphragmatic breathing helps reduce stress.

Our diaphragm is directly connected to our brain via the vagus nerve and the stimulation of this nerve is greatly responsible for our change in state from 'fight and flight' to 'rest and digest' - the two sides of the coin as far as our Autonomous Nervous System goes.

As we spend our days sitting at our desks, working on our laptops, we tend to be performing activities that may cause high levels of arousal - no, I don't mean those kinds of computer based actions… I'm talking about the arousal of our sympathetic nervous system or 'fight and flight' response. We tend to get triggered through the growing and instant demands for our work. If we are taking shallow breaths into our chest this only makes things worse.

BUT - we have the ability to control and reverse this unpleasant and dangerous cycle through use of our breath - or, more specifically, can you guess it… through the use of our diaphragm.

As we breathe in using our diaphragm we trigger the parasympathetic nervous system - or the 'rest and digest' response. The vagus nerve which is the trigger for this strong cue to relax, links the diaphragm directly to the brain. And why shouldn't it? We are inactive (sitting) and therefore in a resting position. By employing the diaphragm and massaging our guts, getting things flowing again and triggering the vagus nerve, it is the best time to be sending signals to the brain to 'rest and digest'.

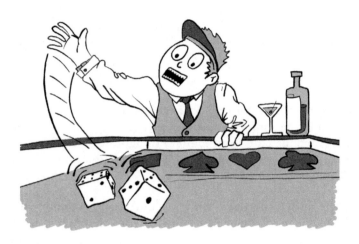

The vagus nerve - not to be confused with 'the Vegas nerve'...

If we are stressed at work, our shallow chest breathing, caused by poor posture, further inhibits both our ability to breathe deeply and to relax through stimulation of the vagus nerve. By simply performing full diaphragmatic breaths, we can take the edge off stress and bring ourselves back, closer to our balance point. These signals override the stress response coming from our restrictive posture and triggering emails to allow us to chill the hell out.

It literally puts us back in the driving seat and helps us chill out - go on - feel into that nice deep 'belly breath' again. Smile, notice how good it feels. Maybe you can notice things slowing down, calming down, feeling that little bit better too. Triggering the vagus nerve also slows down our heartbeat, calming us still further and getting us back to that relaxed feeling we deserve to have when sitting.

Never Missing a Beat with our Heart

While we are speaking of the heart, the diaphragm is also directly connected to the heart. They're pen pals and they have an emergency phone connection. Our diaphragm is quite the busy two-shoes isn't it? There are only a few gaps in the diaphragm and these are to allow our digestive tracts to pass through and also for our major arteries and veins (the vena cava and aorta) to pass through uninhibited to our lower abdomen. But it is also directly linked to the heart through a complex network of nerves.

If we pause and think about both these organ's purposes, it's obvious that they'd be intimately connected. As our diaphragm is our major breathing muscle the diaphragm is the organ best placed to tell the heart how hard to work and vice-versa. The more energy we require the more air we need to take in, and the more blood we need to pump around our body to get that oxygen to the parts that need it most. To cope with this added demand, our airways and blood-vessels also open - or dilate - to allow more air in and blood to move around with minimal effort.

The whole circulatory system is there to help get oxygen to our cells and carbon dioxide out again. We breathe in, oxygen is taken into our blood, the heart pumps it around, it takes the carbon dioxide rich blood back to the lungs and we exhale it out.

The important bit is getting the oxygen to our cells as quickly as we can for as long as we can. With support from a combination of micro-muscles around our artery walls, and vents throughout our cardio-vascular system, we minimise the amount of energy the heart needs to use to pump this blood around. Our breathing is directly linked with this process, working and dancing in perfect harmony. Every time we inhale, our heartbeat increases in speed, and as we exhale, it slows down. We need to work to pump oxygen rich blood, and are then able to relax in-between as we get ready for the next inhale.

As such, in a perfectly healthy body this is easily recognised and in fact this difference is now being used to measure and track athletes' true fitness levels to a higher standard than other methods out there. Have you heard of heart rate variability (HRV) yet? Based on your heart rate and how it varies between the inhale and exhale, this is the difference of how hard the heart works between an in and out breath. The more effective and the greater the variability, the greater the efficiency and therefore the better our' fitness 'level.

We all want and need to look after our heart. We want to take off as much pressure as possible, and our friend the diaphragm is no stranger here either. Nice slow diaphragmatic breathing will lessen the load on the heart and ensure we have many more beats in the bag, translating to plenty more happy days ahead of us.

EXERCISE
Take a Nice Deep Breath or Three

So go on, take another few deep breaths in, just using the diaphragm, and see if you can feel into all these factors at work to keep you healthy and strong.

Can you feel your belly expanding, can you feel the movement of organs in your guts?

Can you feel a wash of calm emanate from your guts to the rest of your body?

And can you feel the difference between the inhale, and, the exhale? The blood, pumping round the body. Feels great doesn't it?!

Chapter 4
The Nose

Everyone now seems finally to be talking about nasal breathing - and that's a very good thing! It's not a passing fad, it's the healthiest and most efficient way to breathe. James Nestor and his excellent bestseller *Breath* from 2020 was the *Supersize Me* for the breathwork world. It rightly took the world by storm and thanks to his work, and the media attention since, nasal breathing has firmly cemented itself on the stage of wellbeing.

Though it may break a lot of preconceived norms and popular misbeliefs, we actually get more air into our lungs by breathing through our nose than we do our mouth, as well as a lot more oxygen into our body. Despite seemingly flying in the face of a logic that suggests we need to dump the waste gas as fast as possible, it is also a lot healthier to also exhale through the nose.

I grew-up in the countryside and was allergic to just about everything. Despite my allergies, I also had an adventurous spirit and would run wild and free every moment I wasn't in school, and to be fair I was a tear-away *in* school too. Whether racing home-made go karts down steep hills, having stick, apple and then later, fire and airgun fights with my friends or building forts in farmers fields, scrumping and cutting down trees, our days were spent outside and I suffered accordingly. All the while my nose would be fully bunged-up at best, my eyes on fire at worst. I suffered more at different times of the year and despite being told I'd grow out of it when I was a teenager, these problems persisted well past my 13th birthday.

I'd get home from staging battles in local corn fields or carving secret tunnels and camps in hay barns and my eyes would be red-raw, I'd be tearing at the flesh around my eyes and my nose would be streaming. The rest of the time I was just plumb bunged-up. I couldn't breathe through my nose even if I wanted to, and I didn't.

For decades my nose was my enemy and if not blocked-up then the internal membranes were inflamed, and would stop all airflow leaving my nose as nothing but some strange triangular thing that stuck out from the middle of my face.

When I first became interested in breathwork for free-diving and scuba, the focus was to consciously slow my heart rate and therefore blood flow, so that I could safely stay under the water for longer. However, because we used snorkels and regulators all this time I kept breathing through my mouth.

My experience with yogic breathing or pranayama, was often met with frustration, anxiety and failure. 'Just relax and breathe in through your nose 'was the constant advice I was getting - despite my insistence that I couldn't. Instructors got annoyed with me and my 'desire to fail', which pushed a few too many of my buttons. After snapping back one time 'I just can't! 'I realised this wasn't too conducive to a yoga practice nor doing any of us any good, so I left never to darken their doors again.

Around the same time I discovered and embraced the Wim Hof Method (WHM) of breathing because, apart from other benefits, it was said you could 'breathe in through any hole'. At last I had found my tribe! However, as information and materials were very thin on the ground back then, I was of course only getting half of the story. As a practice the WHM strongly recommends nasal breathing - but just for the duration of the exercises, it's OK to switch to/use the mouth.

And so, continuing to only breathe through my mouth was adding to my ever growing list of issues, from anxiety and insomnia to binge-eating and drinking. But what to do?

There are millions of people like us out there, but there's hope.

Once I had unlocked the knowledge, thanks mostly to the Buteyko Method and Patrick McKeown's work with The Oxygen Advantage, I was able to not only breathe through my nose properly for the first time, but unlock all those superpowers that everyone else had taken for granted all of their lives.

Hopefully this section will help other sufferers like myself, and also everyone else, to enhance your breathing whether your goals are athletic prowess or just a little less stress in your life - or both, that's OK too.

This has been one of the most difficult things in my life to change and yet, as such, (perhaps because of it) it has been the one that has brought me the most benefits.

Before we dive into the complex roles nasal breathing has, let's first recap on that nice easy way to remember what a good breath is. A nice deep breath. Deep: The furthest from the surface. So a nice deep breath should be in through the nose and deep down into the lower part of our lungs. Not fully extending, not pushing to bursting, just nice and comfortable, nice and deep.

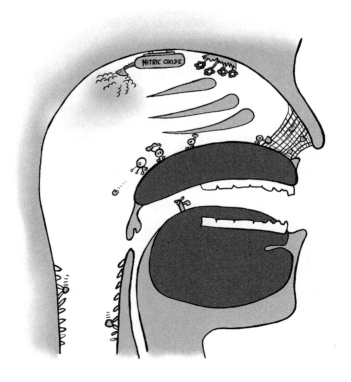

Nose vs mouth breathing: filtration, syphons and added nitric oxide

Nose Holes (Nostrils)

Let's take a look at the structure of the nose. It's got smaller holes than our mouth, so logic dictates that if we want to breathe more easily and more efficiently we should just use the big hole. If it was as simple as that then yes, this would be the case and we would have evolved that way - however, as you may be starting to work out, things are a little bit more complex than just taking air in and out as fast as possible when it comes to breathing.

The small orifices of our nose serve the distinct purpose of slowing down our breath. The deliberate slowing of our breath allows all the other factors involved in each inhale and exhale to come into play. And this is where it gets really fun, interesting and, if you are really getting into this now, somewhat mind blowing!

Watch your Speed

As we inhale, the air enters our nasal passageway which suddenly opens up into a large area, which is shaped like a turbine or conch shell. These turbine like structures are called turbulates and their primary task is to circulate the air and allow it to mix properly in our nasal cavity, and align itself so that the air goes smoothly down through our neck (actually our trachea and bronchi) and into our lungs. This means that even a sharp inhale through the nose enters down into our lungs in a nice smooth flow.

Don't just take my word for it. Go on. Give it a try!

If we take a sharp inhalation in through our mouth, the air shoots directly backwards, hitting the back of our mouth and throat before being forced to sharply turn direction to go down into our lungs - over time this causes all kinds of problems from tracheal trauma to increased infections, tooth decay and bad breath.

Breathing in through the mouth is connected to and directly stimulates chest breathing. Viewed horizontally, instead of a long upside-down capital L or hockey-stick of a relaxed deep nasal breath, the curve of our breath is shorter and more angulated - like a capital C or a boomerang. This means chest breaths will be of the shallow variety, shifting very little fresh air into our lungs.

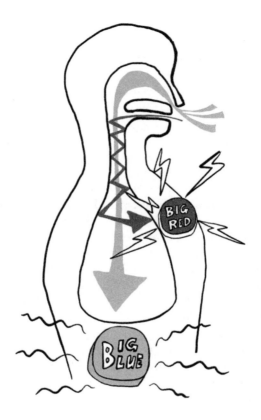

Air Filter

Breathing in at a slower rate also allows us to filter the air more effectively. Our nose hairs and cilia perform the vital task of catching any larger particulates (eg: dust or pollen) that might be in the air we breathe, and the layers of mucus attached to them help to catch that stuff before it gets into our lungs. Have you ever sat around a campfire, gone on a dusty hike or spend a day near busy roads and then blown your nose? I bet you freaked-out at how black your snot was. Well, at least it's all there caught in your bogies than inhaled deep down into our precious little alveoli in our lungs!

More problematic particles are also caught and filtered out in the mucus at other stages during our inhalation and these can be harmlessly drawn down into the fiery hell of our stomach acid to be disposed of safely, or hawked back up like a premier league footballer. It's the same important result though - this stuff doesn't get into our lungs where the damage is done, unlike with mouth breathing.

Award Winning Drugs

As the air is drawn into our nose and circulated around nicely, it also mixes with nitric oxide (NO) - which is produced in the sinuses at ten times the levels than can be found in the mouth. Now, this shouldn't be confused with nitrous oxide (NOX) or laughing gas, which has no benefits except to give you a hell of a head-rush, as it kills brain cells on a professional level and litters the streets with bullet shaped canisters...

Nitric oxide is an absolute legend of a gas. In the 1990s it even won its own Nobel Prize but it's still not classified on the Periodic Table as a noble gas...

Anyway, moving swiftly on:

Dr Furchgott, Ignarro and Murad won this prestigious award when they identified the previously unknown health benefits it carries. A breath rich in nitric oxide will relax and open up airways from our bronchioles in our neck, all the way down to our lovely little air sacs the alveoli. This means that more air (or oxygen) is able to be inhaled and delivered to where it is needed with less effort - meaning an even more effective and efficient breath.

Oh, but it doesn't stop there! Nitric Oxide also helps open up our blood vessels meaning greater and more efficient blood flow. This aids us in all kinds of interesting and genuinely fun ways. From increased absorption of Oxygen in our alveoli to greater blood flows to our extremities, it also greatly helps with circulation issues and is also the major effective ingredient in

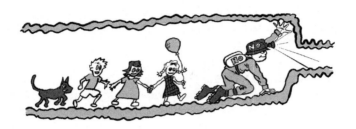

Nitric oxide acts as a dilator,
opening both our airways and blood vessels

Viagra and other similar medications…

Note: rather than reach for a blue pill to help 'circulation issues', why not eat more nitrogen rich foods instead and let the body do what it does best? Beetroot and pomegranate juice have been tested on athletic performance - on the track, not between the sheets - with very promising results. Can we breathe for better sports performance and better sexual prowess with the same results? Popular thinking is a resounding, 'Yes'.

Wet and Warm

Who's seen a dog on a hot day? What are they doing? OK - yes, apart from rolling around in smelly puddles, trying to hump everything and hilariously refusing to come back to their human companions despite their frantic shouts!

Maybe I should be a bit more specific… On a hot day, relating to their breathing, what do dogs do?

They pant. Their tongue lolls out of their mouth and they pant. And why do dogs pant? Because they can't sweat and this is the next best way to lose heat and moisture. Warm air moves over the moist tissues of lungs, throat and lastly the lolling tongue in their mouth, taking the heat energy with each breath as it leaves their bodies.

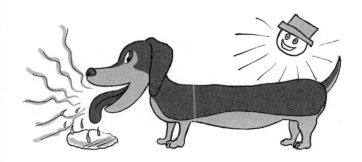

A hot dog. Panting allows for heat loss through evaporation.

Water needs a lot of energy to warm it up. To warm water to a level where it changes from a liquid to a gas that can be exhaled, takes a *lot* of energy. The form of energy used here is heat. Simply put, this means the exhaler can - and has - lost a lot of body heat. It's super efficient and it's the way our canine friends have evolved. (Admittedly yes, the other is to jump, lie and bask in muddy puddles, but we're looking at breathing here. For the health benefits of mud baths look to *Mud Baths, the clinical case* by Dr Muddy McMudFace. An excellent read).

Like dogs, when we pant or mouth-breathe we can get rid of unwanted heat but, we also lose moisture. Unlike dogs, we can sweat. We have evolved far more efficient ways to cool ourselves naturally and if we resort to panting to lose heat we can quickly find ourselves in danger. In everyday situations and exertions, panting for humans is simply not advised.

NOTE: If we are overly hot and we are not sweating, then we may have already entered into the more dangerous level of heat exhaustion/heatstroke, in these such situations please seek emergency help or interventions immediately.

Breathing through the mouth has exactly the same effect on heat and water loss as panting, just to a lesser degree. One of the end products of cell metabolism (remember that fun, long equation?) is water. If we have an excess of water, as well as urination we exhale it back out. When we are mouth-breathing we have no control over the amount of water we are exhaling. This loss can build-up considerably and can push us from mild dehydration to a more severe case on normal days, but especially so when the mercury in the thermometer starts to rise.

Looking back, it is no wonder that I often found it hard to concentrate and would get overly tired mid-morning and afternoon - sometimes feeling like I just needed to fall asleep. I was constantly in trouble at school for yawning all morning and then dismissed as 'one of those students 'at uni for the same reason (admittedly, by that point, I was' one of those students ' but that's by the by).

Through my mouth breathing I was not only taking shallow and inefficient breaths, leading to lower metabolism and brain fog, I was also losing too much moisture simply through my breathing pattern. Combine this with too much coffee and alcohol in my diet and it left me feeling slow, uncomfortable and led to a greater number of headaches than my similarly heavy-drinking friends. I was also dehydrated. Just like low levels of oxygen and food, water is absolutely essential for every process in the human body and for life itself. It's not something we want to unknowingly lose.

At the time, I put this down to my lifelong allergies and 'weaker disposition 'but now it is as clear as day. I could have reversed these harmful trends, that only got worse as I got older, by following that simple advice, often yelled at me in primary school:

'Gus Hoyt - would you for once just shut your mouth?!'

Studies have found that we lose 42% more moisture breathing through our mouth, than through our nose. (Svensson, Olin and Hellgren 2006). This is a lot and shouldn't be dismissed. The NHS advice is drinking between six and eight cups of water a day and more if pregnant or breastfeeding, in a hot environment, physically active for long periods or ill or recovering from illness. We definitely need to add 'and if you're breathing through your mouth 'onto this list too.

As we exhale through our nose, the air exits through those conch shell-shaped turbulates again, coming into contact with our fleshy insides and due to a slower pace to the air, it is 'caught 'held and reabsorbed far more effectively at this stage. When air-bound water is channelled into a smaller volume it is compressed together. This forces the water molecules in gas form, into contact with each other and these form larger water droplets. These droplets (and the clue is in the name) are heavier than the air and 'drop 'back down onto the surface below and are reabsorbed by our body. The funnel of the nose acts as a condensation chamber and through breathing out of our nose as well as in, we stop our breath from stealing our precious body water.

You can really feel this too if you are new to nasal breathing when jogging - there are other factors at play too but the first thing you'll notice is that your nose just won't stop running! This phenomenon passes quickly as the body soon adapts, but it catches us by surprise at first! This is because we are still breathing the volumes of air we would when mouth breathing but forcing it through these two little condensation channels, turning the taps to flow full pace!

HEATWAVE TIP: A really important trick as we head into an ever warming world, with more frequent heatwaves and while our cities still remain unprepared, is to *slow down*. Moving more slowly, but also slowing our breath right down. Breathing calmly through our nose will both serve to keep us calmer, and also help us to maintain our water levels and stave off dehydration and heatstroke. Of course we need to drink more water but incorporating a healthy breathing pattern is also key.

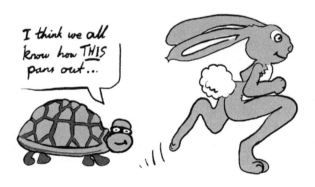

Slow and Steady Wins the Race

Why is fast breathing or mouth breathing really such a bad thing? If oxygen is what we need for energy then we want to breathe in more air right? How can breathing in *more air* really be that bad a thing?

Let's roll it back a little further again and think of the basics of *why we breathe* in the first place, and how breathing through the nose can help us to get more of what we need.

We breathe so that our bodies can take in oxygen which is used in cell metabolism - to create the energy we need for life itself - and to get rid of the by-product of carbon dioxide.

We inhale, the air goes into our lungs, the oxygen passes down the various branches of our lungs to the alveoli, where it passes over a semi-permeable membrane and enters our bloodstream. At the same time, carbon dioxide exits our blood into the now empty alveoli and we breathe this back out into the world beyond.

If we imagine the blood supply - our red blood cells - as buses again, they pull-up at the station, passengers get off and on and then the bus departs full of eager commuters ready to get on with their job at hand.

Perfect!

If we are breathing too fast - if those buses arrive at the depot and instead of slowing down, they keep charging through at 60mph, then we create that familiar feeling of frustration as we miss the bus and need to wait for the next one. We can't get to the office and the work piles-up on our desks... But then the next bus screams past at 60mph as well and soon we have a backlog of workers with no way to leave the station. We have a complete system-jam: gridlock.

In our body, when we over-breathe, what is happening is that we are taking in more than we need too. That is, we are taking in air at a greater pace than our body's demand is for oxygen. At the same time we exhale out too much, or all of our carbon dioxide. We 'dump 'carbon dioxide. When the oxygen-packed red blood cells come along, the haemoglobin bond isn't broken as there's no carbon dioxide to do this task.

The result is the red blood cells carry-on being pumped around our body by our heart fully ladened with oxygen. The transfer of oxygen to the cells is blocked and the primary objective of breathing is thwarted.

Despite breathing *more* or *faster,* we are actually unable to get the oxygen we need to where it needs to go. The system is collapsing and panic sets-in as our hungry cells cry out for more!

Herein lies a deeper problem. When our cells cry for more we trigger the stress process and this opens-up the body to take in *more air* and ironically favours *faster* breathing, *shallower* breathing and *mouth* breathing - the holy trifecta of what NOT to do in this situation! This is a strange abnormality in our body, and one that used to confuse me. At the time we most need to slow our breathing down, our body is triggered into doing just the opposite and this can have harmful short, and disastrous long term results.

For effective gaseous exchange to happen, and this is why we breathe after all, we need to slow down our breaths, especially in stressful situations. We need to take deeper breaths and this means in through the nose and deep down, using the diaphragm, thus filling our lower lungs before our chest. We need efficient slower breaths, so correct gaseous exchange can take place.

Blocked Nose

But what if we still can't breathe through our nose? What if, for whatever reason we physically or psychologically can't? For decades I thought and believed through my whole being that I couldn't breath in through my nose. Due to allergies, internal swelling and a lifetime of learning this 'truth', I simply couldn't do it. Any attempt would lead to frustration and anger, and this would trigger my stress response, making things even harder still - so I DO get it if you say you can't, but bear with me.

There may be many reasons we suffer from blocked noses, and I would suggest seeing a specialist if you genuinely cannot breathe through your nose. That said, I saw specialists for the first two decades of my life to no avail and respite only came when I started consciously making baby steps to improve my breathing, by focusing on my breathing rather than on what was wrong with me.

My breathing is still far from perfect, but the improvements I have seen have turned my life around. So it's certainly worth investing a little time every day.

There are lots of simple exercises later in the book (skip ahead if you need them) that we can use to open up our airways, balance our systems within and find that golden state of homeostasis, where everything starts working again as it should.

However if you are feeling blocked-up and/or have always struggled breathing here's a great one from the book 'The Oxygen Advantage' that I have adapted and like to call:

EXERCISE
The Nodder

- Inhale and exhale normally
- Pinch your nose and breathe very gently into the cavity around your nose (like you do trying to acclimatise on an aeroplane)
- As you gently exhale into this space nod very deliberately - but not head-banging
- Nod 5-20 times or whenever you feel a need to breathe again
- Let go of your nose and slowly inhale through it Breath 'normally 'for about 30 seconds and then Repeat five times

Each time you'll find that the nasal passageways open a little more (you probably won't feel it but your bronchioles and alveoli will open a little more too, due to the release of the extra pooled nitric oxide) DO repeat five times though. Don't just stop as soon as you feel that they have opened. This can be performed pretty much anywhere and will bring respite within no time. You cannot repeat this exercise too many times.

You'll even overcome your inhibitions about doing this in a public place, once you start to really feel the benefits of nasal over mouth breathing!

Normal Nose Swelling

Swelling of the inside of our nose is normal - and strangely one nostril will always be slightly more blocked (or open) than the other. This operates in a cycle of around 40-45 minutes. Why do you think this might be?

Apply all you have read already here so far and have a little think about the practical applications of this.

There's always an answer because everything happens in the body for a reason, everything is interconnected.

Here's another picture for you to look at, if your thought processes are more visually stimulated.

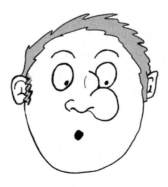

And have you found an answer - a theory - something that could be tested in a lab?

Fantastic - then get hold of a lab and see if they will be interested in testing your hypothesis - as this is just one of those things that we still just don't know yet! This is still one of those great unsolved mysteries - and that's pretty exciting really because there are so few left in the world today - especially concerning something right in front of our face!

There are lots of theories and the most frequently put forward comes from the pranayama and yogic practices, which states that nasal breathing stimulates different parts of our body and that breathing in through the left nostril feeds the right side of our brain, which in turn stimulates creativity and promotes calm, while breathing in through the right nostril brings warmth into the body and stimulates the left side of the brain and the logic/problem-solving processes.

There are many conscious techniques you can use to benefit either your creativity or concentration, etc and this shouldn't be confused with alternate nostril breathing, known as Nadī Shodhana in Sanskrit which has many proven benefits. But we just don't know why the body switches from one nostril to the other every 40 minutes or so. Or maybe we do and science just hasn't caught up yet. I'm going to leave that one hanging.

And so there you have it, for very good reasons, everyone and their dog is raving about nasal breathing at the moment, but unlike so many health trends out there it's not a fad. This is a mainstay and foundation for healthy breathing and a healthy life. So, no matter how difficult it may be, start your journey to becoming a nose breather once and for all. If you really do struggle then why not jump on the Oxygen Advantage website and find a coach near you who can help guide you on your own personal journey? There's a free app too - but like all apps, it can only really be used in combination with a good teacher.

From increased uptake of oxygen to losing less water from our bodies, from filtering out impurities to smoothing the air flow for maximum absorption, our noses play a tonne of important roles - and some are still yet to be discovered! How fun is that?!

And we haven't even fully explored the effects on stress control yet.

Chapter 5
Stress and the Nervous System

Stress is, in and of itself, not a bad thing. It's one of those catch-all phrases that is used far too readily and loosely. As with everything in life, simply thinking of things as good or bad is unhelpful at best, harmful at worst and the same is true of our perception of 'stress' and the purposes it serves.

We have evolved alongside stress and it's safe to say it has saved our neck millions of times over. In fact, we could say that we are all here today because all our past ancestors had effective stress responses. It gets us out of immediate danger and over time it helps us to avoid it in the first place. It can give us almost superhuman abilities, which can save our skin and perform amazing feats of survival. In recent years, we have even found that deliberately embracing very stressful activities can 'reboot ' and strengthen the systems within the body, through harnessing the benefits that these positive stressors (or 'eustress') brings.

But on the flip-side, stress is also the number one killer in the 'western world'. So where do we go with this?!

Let's unpack this a little bit and ask ourselves about the relationship between stress and breathing. After all, that's what we're here to talk about. To do so we're going to have to investigate what we mean by stress, the different kinds, the effects it has on our body, the relationship with our breath and ultimately, how we *can control* our stress response with our breath alone.

But first let's look at stress in our daily lives - how it affects us now, today.

Take a few nice slow deep breaths and feel into your body. Stop reading. Put the book down, and take three slow, deep breaths.

Now cast your mind back to the last time you opened your emails and saw a really triggering message. One you likely avoided opening, as you didn't feel like you could deal with it then and there for whatever reason. Think about the last time you were unexpectedly called to speak in a public meeting or when your behaviour was challenged by a loved one. How did that make you feel?

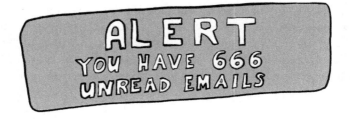

How we feel and what goes on in our body are intrinsically linked. In fact how we feel is our way of simplifying and coding of what's happening in our body - based on past experiences and outcomes both real and imaginary. They are short-cuts so we don't have to make a thousand decisions each time the scenario arises. We *feel* what we need to do and 'instinctively 'do it.

Let's think back to that feeling - that response, the rising stress and how it manifested in the body and what it felt like. Our heart rate increases, our breathing becomes shallow, more chest-orientated. As adrenaline is released into our system, blood-flow is redirected away from our guts and the higher, cerebral parts of the brain and towards our muscles, which need to be ready for action but which may shake or twinge uncontrollably. Our senses are heightened and time seems to slow down. We may feel a rush of energy - perhaps as misdirected heat or a flushed face.

All in all, it doesn't feel nice and if we're already feeling stressed, or threatened, then this just adds to the unpleasantness of the feeling. Often we sweat, go red, shake or even start to panic a little. In most modern situations, we become more self-conscious, our inner critic raises its voice and we start to feel very uncomfortable. This adds the perceived threat to our safety and ramps-up our stress response still further. Things feel even worse and we spiral out of control.

Our stress response is hindering, rather than serving us. But this is more a problem caused by the modern world than by our ancient bodily systems themselves.

So what's it all about? Why would our bodies react like this?

First off we need to remember that we are animals which have evolved over millions of years. We are now living in a fast-changing and unnatural world of our making to which we have not yet naturally adapted.

As we're no longer living in natural conditions, it should be no surprise at all that our evolutionary stress response is a little out of sync with our daily needs. It has served us so well throughout history and will again, following the collapse of civilisation as we know it, but for now it's dancing to a different beat.

Stress is generally labelled as the 'fight or flight 'response. Danger is often simplified to the exaggerated example of confronting a bear in the wild - we can either fight it or run away. (Let's not get into the standing ground vs running and brown bears vs black bear debate here…). To punch or to run? Again, a simple choice that doesn't serve us all that well in most day to day scenarios…

Our stress response evolved for survival. We are animals. Plain and simple. When we feel threatened, it kicks in, adrenaline is released, our heart pumps more blood faster around the body. Energy is released and muscles are prepped and readily able to gobble it all up. Our higher brain functions are put on hold and our senses sharpen, as we focus on the threat at hand. In today's world we are often in no actual physical danger but the response is still the same.

That triggering email is a signal of threat and it starts the process to prepare our body to respond to this danger. As we interpret this as *real* danger, this naturally affects both our feelings and wellbeing. We also have no way to reduce this building adrenaline in our body, we've not fought-off the bear or run away - unless you have of course, but apparently that's not acceptable in an office environment.

Our actions are then at loggerheads with what our body has been primed to do. This creates a *huge* disconnect and an internal clash. We are left feeling uncomfortable, dreadful and close to collapse. We are literally full of unfulfilled potential and it's even more tiring to suppress it until the adrenalin runs out, leaving us feeling exhausted.

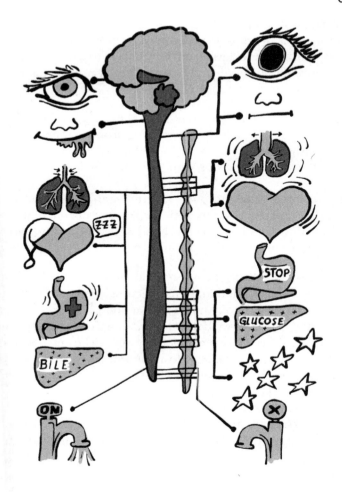

Split into two, the parasympathetic and the sympathetic nervous systems.
The PNS dilates our eyes, stimulates saliva, slows the heart and breathing rate, increases stomach activity and the production of bile and relaxes our bladder.
The SNS constricts our pupils, stops saliva and stomach activity, increases our heart and breath rate, releases glucose and adrenaline and shuts off our bladder.

Our Nervous Systems

Our nervous systems have evolved to pass information and feedback from our external and internal environments back and forth through our body and brain. Without it we wouldn't last a moment even in the nicest of places.

Our central nervous system (CNS) is the one we think of most, and this is responsible for everything from us being able to consciously move our bodies, whether it is to play a piano concerto or to dance along with Gangnam Style.

Information is passed through electrical impulses in our nerve-structures and also saves us from danger, leaping out of the way of a speeding car or pulling our hand away from a burning pan before we even have time to think about it.

The aspect we are most concerned about is a lesser, but just as vital strain called the autonomic nervous system (ANS) which operates all those bodily functions we don't have time to think about, and if we did we'd lack the time to make even the most basic of life-decisions. From blood pressure to bowel movement, our ANS takes care of it all. Most importantly for us here today though, it also maintains our breathing and heart rates. We just breathe, it's taken care of 20,000 times a day.

Micro-stressors and Triggers

We are triggered by SO many aspects of our daily lives, from missed calls to messages that haven't been sent, from the alert on our phones to an email inbox, from a lack of social media likes to a confrontation in the workplace, be it over our washing-up etiquette or our monthly performance review. All these things can and do trigger a stress response - no way near as large as if a grizzly bear charged towards you knocking desks and family photos asunder, intent on gnawing on your bones - but stress responses nonetheless.

Over time these smaller stressors build on each other. Small events that cause us stress, but don't fully engage a stress response slowly build-up over the day and end up wearing us out. These so-called micro-stressors can come in many guises and estimates of how many we have a day, vary wildly depending on classification. More conservative studies demonstrate we can experience around 50 of these a day, others are in the thousands.

Though released into the body at great speed, the adrenaline in our body takes longer to dissipate. After the initial surge it can take at least twenty minutes for the adrenalin to dissipate and us to start to return to 'normal 'again, longer if the stressor remains. This means that the adrenalin is left to either slowly dissipate out of our system or, as in most workplaces today, build and build as the day wears-on. This leads us into a continued state of low-level stress and is not only common, but it is seen by health practitioners as a pandemic of the modern workplace/life. This is chronic stress and it *is* a killer.

But there *is* good news! We can control this process, and by being more aware and in control of our breath is the key to freedom we desire. Before we look at exactly how though, let's explore what is going on in the body first.

Why Did we Develop the Stress Response?

So what is the stress response, and if it's good for us, why does it feel so bad and why is it 'the number one killer 'in the West?

Evolutionary Aspects:

We have evolved, and are alive today, in part because those who came before us had an effective stress response. They were able to react to danger in a way that meant they survived long enough to reproduce. We are animals and have developed a complex 'fight or flight 'response that means that when faced with dangers our ancestors either fought that bear or they ran away from it.

This worked well when we were living wild and free but over time, and especially during the last couple of hundred of years, we have deliberately placed ourselves and our lives outside of the natural world and order of things. Rarely do we see a wild bear anymore, and if we do it's probably from the safety of a 4x4 or we have a gun or pepper-spray to protect us. Yet, we still face real danger and threats and we still have this innate but basic response for us to deal with these threats.

A Modern 'Bear Attack'

Let's look at this in a more modern context. Almost a decade ago it was yet another repressively humid day in New Orleans. Despite it being almost Christmas - or perhaps because of it, all my friends and work colleagues had gone home and the restaurant was closed for the Twixmas period. After rummaging around my apartment I managed to gather the $4.98 needed for a six-pack of cheap beer and momentary solace.

Walking down Burgundy Street in the French Quarter I met a man with a gun blocking my path. I was exhausted, depressed and self-absorbed, now there was some stranger waving a gun trying to get into my world…

My assailant was met with incredulation, bemusement and then outright disregard at the fact he was robbing me. *Me*, who worked his ass-off for little over minimum wage, and who had to search for loose change just to be able to buy some crap beer! My mugger started to panic and stopped waving the gun around and pointed it in my face.

He told me to stop messing around and take off my shoes in case that's where I was hiding the money.

I was negotiating with him, explaining my situation, how I was poor. In no time, I was talking at a million miles an hour. It had recently rained and my socks got wet. I was *pissed* off. I started to get really angry - but still handed over the money.

'Next time rob a rich f***ing tourist!' I yelled after him.

My legs then turned to jelly and I collapsed.

An interesting thing had happened - apart from my near death experience. It had taken ages for my adrenalin to kick-in. It felt like hours, but at the time was probably only a minute or so.

A little while later, someone checked on me and lent me their phone to call the police. Not that I really had much to report, in a city like New Orleans, one small mugging was hardly a police priority but I thought I had better call it in all the same. Cue a very surreal hour, where I became the centre of a CSI episode. It turned out that they were in the middle of a sting on robberies on tourists and my accent put me in that category (Queen's English).

What had happened here? It took a while but my frustration and disappointment quickly turned to anger and rage and then I had collapsed.

My body had experienced an incredibly strong fight or flight response but it took a few minutes. The threat of a gun seemed alien to me, and so it didn't trigger the emergency signals in my brain it does now. Then, due to the severity of the situation, the adrenalin really kicked-in. Higher brain functions were muted and I got angry and argued with a guy with a gun… Afterwards, coupled with the fact I hadn't really slept in months (#ChefLife), I discovered the other aspect of this 'survival 'reaction and *freeze* came into play. My body burnt through all available energy and then, like a possum, my body just 'died'.

When I realised my man was serious and wasn't backing down, I had wanted to fight the guy - thank god I didn't try - and then this turned to rage and lock-down. Not the best response when confronted with a gun, but then we haven't evolved yet to deal with guns, no matter what the Hollywood action movies might suggest. Perhaps we shall evolve into higher cognitive powers that let us negotiate our way out, but I hope guns aren't a central part of our culture for much longer.

What may - or may not - have worked on the bear was prescribed for this situation too. Maybe I would have been shot if I'd fought, but then if you try and fight a bear you'd certainly lose too. I didn't run for some reason, but I did collapse.

This is the third leg of the stool fight, flight and freeze - evolutionarily it could have helped as the bear may have tossed me around for a bit, hurting but not killing me and my mugger would have been able to go through my pockets (and shoes) before departing, hopefully leaving me similarly 'unharmed'. Like it or lump it, freezing and not fighting had saved my life, as it had evolved to do.

Danger = Stress = Action

Chemical and Physiological Aspects:
So what on earth was going on in my body at the time? All kinds of crazy things is the answer. I was also physically and emotionally drained from a brutal few weeks catering for the pre-Christmas crowd, and drinking too much to 'bring myself' down again after my late finishes. But, let's look at what happened and transpose a perfect stress response over the top to see if we can make sense of it.

I saw the guy blocking my way, he issued his threat and pulled a big gun on me. These messages (finally) made their way through my eyes and ears into the amygdala - an area of the brain tasked with prioritising incoming information based on memory - and sent the 'shit's happening 'signals to my hypothalamus - the command centre - and from here all the Big Red Buttons were pushed!

The hypothalamus is in charge of all the 'involuntary 'functions in our body, all the functions that if we had to sit and think about doing we'd be little more use than a sea cucumber - breathing, digestion, heartbeats, blood pressure and so forth.

Our ANS is split into two wings - the sympathetic and parasympathetic. The fight and flight and the rest and digest elements we know so well. (A commonly used analogy for the two is of an accelerator pedal in a car and the brake pedal - things are of course a LOT more complex than this.)

When, in my case, the hypothalamus hit the Big Red Button for the fight/flight response the sympathetic nervous system came to the forefront, overriding and suppressing the parasympathetic and taking control.

Our adrenal glands hear the call and dump adrenaline (norepinephrine) into our bloodstream. Norepinephrine is both a hormone and a neurotransmitter - this means it affects both our body and brain. We associate adrenaline with something that makes us stronger and this is true, but it's more complex and interesting than that alone.

First off, norepinephrine is a neurotransmitter, that means it sends *fast* messages to the brain. Instantly, we become more alert and aware of our immediate surroundings, our senses become super-tuned and our higher brain functions are suppressed because, well, who needs to do algebra right now?!

While being mugged and confronted by a gun, it took a while to register, but as soon as it did, I was snapped out of my depressed state, brought into the present moment, stopped my 'clever negotiations 'and was hyper-aware of everything going on.

A few moments later, the blood-based adrenaline kicks in. This takes a bit longer, as hormones move around the body in the blood flow and this isn't as immediate as the electric synapses of our brain. The adrenalin does 'make us stronger 'but it does so by giving us a kind of turbo charge or nitro boost.

Glucose is released into our blood. along with dense energy stores of fat, our airways and blood vessels dilate and open to allow more air and blood to flow and our heart beats faster - pumping all the good stuff to where it needs to go. The glucose and oxygen are the fuel and the dial is turned-up to eleven. We get a huge flood of excess energy, which can then be used in the short term by our muscles to either fight the foe at hand or run for the hills!

This also gives us the 'superhuman strength 'often reported in life-threatening situations, such as a mother ripping a car door off its hinges to rescue her children. If the threat is perceived to remain, the hypothalamus also triggers the release of the chemicals cortisol releasing factor (CRH) and adrenocorticotropic hormone (ACTH) which maintain the intensity of our reaction, by releasing higher levels of cortisol long after the initial adrenalin is 'depleted'.

As soon as I was mugged, my shoes removed and the transaction finalised, the threat then disappeared. The gun went back into baggy jeans and the assailant slipped down a side street and immediately out of sight. I wobbled there for a moment, energy surging through my body but unable to process it. Overwhelmed by my near-death experience my legs turned to jelly.

Despite my body giving way, my nervous energy stayed with me. This would have happened for a few reasons but most noticeably that adrenaline stays in our system for a while, just think back to the last time you tried to rationalise with someone who was irate. It just doesn't 'go in'. Add to this the fact that there was no *action*; I didn't fight and even though I could have set a new land-speed record, I didn't run away.

This cocktail of powerful emergency chemicals stayed in my system and just gave me the jitters instead, until I became the bane of the New Orleans Police Department. NOPD officers came to interview me and I turned into a mains-spout of verbal diarrhoea.

Emotional Aspects:

The amygdala - the area of the brain that sensed danger and told my body to react, is a complex little almond-shaped cluster of cells in the base of our brain. This part of our brain stores and processes memories to help us survive. We have evolved to be able to associate and remember dangerous situations, to such an extent that we can also start to recognise potential threats *before* the bear attacks us. This has evolved into a sensitive and fine tuned stress response system that can easily be triggered by these stored memories as emotions.

We don't always have to 'see 'the danger but we sense or 'feel ' it and this can prepare the body ready for action. Without going too deeply into the debate about the cause and role that emotions play, they are the way we *feel* and they are based on both real and imagined situations in our lives. They perform an evolutionary process - not just in fight and flight but also in group dynamics and the passing on of our genes.

I interpreted this initially as rage, when the adrenaline really kicked in - remembering past infractions and bullies - a need to lash out and protect myself, but this soon gave way to a feeling of vulnerability and, with it a great sense of being sad and alone. Following the police adventure I sat on the pavement under a streetlight and cried. When I was done, I did the only thing left, as all my friends were with family and out of town, I went to one of my local bars and for the price of my story I was soon bolstered-up with free drinks and cheery faces. Boosted by that magic of false camaraderie fuelled by cheap booze and loneliness at Christmas.

Not a Bear or Mugger but a Boss

However, an armed mugger in a dark street is luckily about as removed from our daily lives as a bear attack, or the need to fight off that mythical sabre-tooth tiger people on the internet always talk about. This was an example of extreme stress and real danger. It was literally a matter of life and death, despite my not quite realising it at the time.

Realistically though, how many of these situations do we face in a lifetime? Luckily, the answer for the average person is 'not many' or 'none'. But that doesn't mean that we don't face high stakes, stressful confrontations on a regular basis. In fact we are most likely dealing with greater stress demands today, than those faced by our caveman forebears.

What *real life* situations can we compare this to? Sadly there are far too many overly stressful situations and confrontations in our daily lives - from the overbearing boss to the pressures we put on ourselves, due to advertising and unrealistic demands like body-image and the accumulation of wealth.

But let's look at that modern ogre or bear. The modern threat most of us deal with on a regular basis is our boss. Even for those who are self-employed, as Bob Dylan said. *We all gotta serve somebody* '- we all have/or have had a boss at some point.

(On an aside - I've always found it pretty interesting that in video game parlance we call the arch nemesis - the end of level baddie that we need to destroy or overcome a 'Boss 'or the 'loss-level'.)

So, our bosses, our supervisors, our team-leaders are a consistent source of stress both real and imagined. Let's look at direct confrontation - that 'meeting about an elapsed deadline', that chat over coffee about targets not getting hit, a client lost or complaints from customers.

The fear of losing our job, of then missing rent or mortgage payments, or losing our partner or children is all very real indeed. In these situations, and apart from all the constant micro-stressors we continually face in the workplace, these events can trigger a response just as strong as the proverbial bear attack or being confronted with a mugger.

These are our everyday modern day bear attacks and *exactly the same* thing happens to us inside.

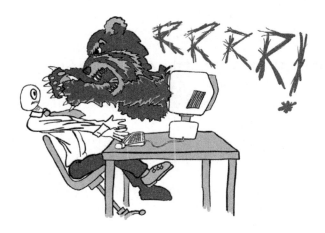

In our workplaces, an added pressure is applied to us though and one that can have long term negative side effects. Though the 'fight/flight response 'firmly kicks in, we aren't allowed or able to run away or fight our way out of the situation. Obviously, some do and these people, like me, have a long and varied employment CV, but most of the time we have to actively *suppress* it!

But, we *can* do something about it to help ourselves. It's super simple and can be done anywhere, anytime we feel the rising pressure of stress.

You've guessed it - take a nice deep breath! Even just taking three slow and deep breaths can make all the difference, reducing stress and panic, returning focus and calm and bringing us back into the driving seat, if possible. If you know you are about to be going into the lion's den, then you can pre-empt the physiological changes and head them off at the pass by starting a slow, calming breathing routine *before a* confrontational situation arises.

But how does this work? Also, how can we control it and what are the consequences if we just let things continue on without intervention?

Stress Breathing and the Adrenaline Rush

We're already realising that an awful lot happens when we breathe, and there's a whole lot more for us still to uncover. When it comes to stress, and the effect on our breath, it's been discovered to work both ways. By taking control of our breath we will soon gain control of our stress response and how it affects us.

We are triggered, a message is sent by the hypothalamus to release adrenaline, which is both a hormone travelling through the blood and a neurotransmitter directly affecting the brain. As a hormone, its job is to get us ready for action by increasing blood-flow and energy release so that our muscles are able to meet the threat head-on.

As our heart rate increases, to pump more blood around the body, we also need to take in more oxygen to fuel that energy exchange. We need to start taking BIG full breaths to meet what our body thinks is a huge immediate demand. We start incorporating the chest and secondary breathing muscles, maybe even the tertiary ones to completely max-out our breath.

The neurotransmitters ensure only the parts of the brain required for immediate survival are operating, and higher functions are restricted in favour of our reaction times and primary senses. Our higher thoughts aren't important at this stage. In the workplace this can leave us on really unstable ground. Our brains are 'frazzled', we can't think straight and we forget common words. All this leads to frustration and fuels the fire that started things in the first place.

In most working environments today, etiquette means we can't bop our boss on the nose or leap out of the window. This throws our stress response out of sync with our immediate and very real needs. As such, this actually ends up doing us even more harm.

Unless we are dealing with physical stress caused by real physical danger, the chances are that we will immediately try to suppress this urge/our need to take big full breaths. What would it look like in the boardroom if we suddenly started massively over-breathing? If we start taking large and audible breaths, panting in an 'aggressive 'manner, chances are the outcome will be almost as bad for us as if we had just run out of the room.

When we get stuck talking to, or being talked at, by our boss or a challenging colleague, we are unable to utilise the energy that's released around our body. This can further exacerbate how we are feeling. The nervous energy is incongruous with what our instinct tells us we should be doing. This disconnect causes us further internal conflict and discomfort. We feel uncomfortable, sad or angry, we feel overwhelmed with frustration and generally just feel terrible.

Most of the time our only outlet is to cry alone in the toilets after work, or blow off steam with colleagues and strangers over a few beers after work.

But it's the breath we are interested in. A stressed breath is a chest breath, it's a shallow breath and will tend to be through an open mouth. We're getting ready for *action*!

Despite our attempts at maintaining composure, the trigger for our breath is automatic and therefore *out* of our control and so we naturally take faster breaths. As the fight and flight response begins, our chest muscles are engaged to max-out the volume of our breath, but as we fight this urge as best we can, we end-up taking more shallow, frequent and less effective or efficient breaths, using our chest or upper abdomen rather than engaging our whole lungs.

To make matters worse, we are most often triggered at work. Here we find ourself sitting at our desk, thus restricting the freedom of our diaphragm, accidentally favouring shallow chest-breaths and paradox breathing. This leads to us already being agitated or 'stressed 'due to poor breathing practices, before we even begin being bombarded with micro-stressors all day long.

I like to think about this like a room of dominoes, spreading-out in a growing pyramid formation. If we knock over one of the tiles they'll keep on falling, building momentum and intensity as they fall until none are left standing. Or we can take evasive action and start employing some deep belly breaths and take a line of dominos away altogether, stopping the 'inevitable' collapse, and hopefully feeling a bit more energised and focused too.

Long-term Dangers

Without action, interaction or a removal of the danger, this process can get completely out of control and spiral quickly into a full blown panic attack. We sometimes even make things worse by trying to fix them - bottling things up, or taking 'deep breaths' into the chest as my childhood doctor 'taught' me.

To a lesser degree this process also leads to elevated breathing patterns that become increasingly normalised the more we tolerate these daily stressors. This makes our predisposition to 'stress' and panic attacks more sensitive. (We will look at how our breath can halt, reverse and prevent this panic response but first, let's look at what's going on.)

When we are triggered, we start breathing into our chest. This is the sympathetic nervous system kicking in, but as we breathe into the chest if we are ignoring deep, healthy diaphragmatic breaths, our breath becomes out of balance. We soon end-up *only* breathing in a sympathetic way, leaving us in a constant state of fight and flight.

This is where it gets really interesting. As we breathe more into our chest, we press that Big Red Button signalling fight/flight - we are pressing the 'on' button for the sympathetic nervous system. Each breath we take into our chest area is a pressing of this Big Red Button!

By not pushing the Big Blue 'Chill' Button located in our diaphragm we are only escalating things and making them worse.

We start spiralling out of control and our breath starts taking control of us. We begin hyperventilating, anxiety rises or goes through the roof and eventually we start getting panic attacks.

Worst case scenario, we pass out. Though this may sound terrible it's actually just our body's 're-boot 'function and our breathing returns to normal almost immediately. It's basically our brain leaning over and saying '*Have you tried turning it off and on again?*' Like fixing a problem TV, this normally does the trick. This is not so great if we're standing-up or near to any sharp objects, driving or operating heavy machinery, but from a purely respiratory point of view, it's great!

There's a big chicken and egg situation going on here - and this is where it gets *really* interesting - and also very helpful too, if we're conscious of what's going on.

Added together, these multiple micro-stressors combine with genuine threatened feelings caused by emails, social media, work and relationships and conspire against our best interests. They perpetuate the chest breathing pattern, we unconsciously start using our mouth to breath more, our posture suffers as we lose core strength and our breathing gets worse still. As we continue to breathe in a 'stressful way '- mouth, chest - we keep feeding the feeling of a threat as if it never goes away.

This is a dangerous downward spiral, and it's one we all find very difficult to get out of. We only make things worse and add to our overall stress levels, which can exaggerate our harmful but generic coping mechanisms of drinking, taking-drugs and staying up late bingeing TV or social media.

The stress response affects how we breathe but just as powerfully, how we breathe affects our stress response.

This keeps our body in a perpetual state of alert. We are triggered and our breathing adjusts. If we limp from trigger to trigger, we continue to breathe as if in a stressful state and our breathing becomes maladjusted.

This maladjusted breath, or dysfunctional breathing pattern starts to become the norm and we get what is known as paradoxical breathing. This means that every single breath we take is inefficient, counterproductive and causes us harm. Bearing in mind we take around 20,000 breaths a day (a lot more for paradoxical breathers) then this is a lot of cumulative 'bad 'we are doing to our bodies.

We are literally deliberately triggering a low-level stress response during every single waking moment, just through the way we are breathing.

If we keep allowing those dominos to fall, they build momentum and they will keep on falling indefinitely - or until they finally run out, and we don't want to completely run out of dominos!

Taking this learning in hand, we can start to create simple and easy ways to manage stress in our everyday lives using this natural tool: our breath.

As with everything, this often sounds easier than it is. After years of high stress work and burnouts, I struggled with my breathing exercises. Due to a perceived lack of time, a wandering and addled mind, it took many months before I was able to regain control of my breath. I was in a really bad way but I came out of the other side and haven't looked back since. This all sounds super simple, and it is, but that doesn't mean it's easy, especially when we are struggling.

A Note on Trauma: If we have suffered trauma in our lives - and we all have to varying degrees - we may tend to act disproportionally in stressful situations. This is perfectly normal, as our survival instinct may be over-sensitive or too finely tuned, and it's just kicking in a little too over-enthusiastically. We are triggered by something around us and our stress response is put into motion. As it is too strong or exaggerated for that situation, it is seen as a disproportionate response.

If our response to stressful situations is too frequently disproportionate, we will find this counterproductive to our daily lives - it starts to hinder us, hold us back and stop us from being able to grow. In these cases conscious breathwork tools can be used to peel back layers of ourselves and help us to identify and tackle the root cause. However, if serious issues are raised or you feel you want to take things further, unless your breathwork coach is also a professional counsellor or psychiatrist, it's best to seek additional help and guidance elsewhere.

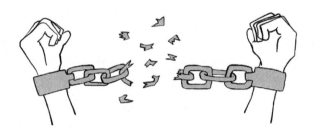

Breaking the Chain

SO, the first thing we are going to do is think back to that perfect deep breath we were talking about earlier. Hopefully by now the learning we covered there has permeated consciously or unconsciously into your daily life.

As we have mentioned, the spread of the stress response and dysfunctional breathing is like the falling of dominos - and just as such, we are able to reach down at any stage and remove a domino or two from the line, thus breaking the pattern and stopping the whole process short.

'All 'we need to do when we start feeling that rise of anxiety is three simple steps:

• Stop what we are doing

- Notice how we are breathing - judgement free
- Slowly move the breath to our belly using the diaphragm alone

And Breathe!

Simple eh? Try it next time you notice you are starting to feel stressed or that your tolerance levels are wavering. I call this my 'Old Faithful'. If you would like a full guided description of this exercise, skip ahead to the final section and you'll find it there amongst some other favourites of mine.

There are a million exercises out there to help. Most focus on counting how long we breathe in and out for. Many of them are excellent and there's a simple selection at the end of this book, but for the most part, following this simple three-step program will help bring balance to your nervous system, reduce stress, pull you back from the edge and help you be far more efficient, effective and happy in your daily life.

The more you practise this exercise the more you will also discover the ability to attune with yourself. This is one of the greatest powers of breathwork and will be covered in more detail later. Put simply it is the ability to really *listen* to your body and understand what it is you really *need* or need to do.

Keeping in the theme of threes, here are three more aspects you can build into this practice, so that you aren't just fire-fighting but starting to build a healthy and holistic approach to your everyday breathing:

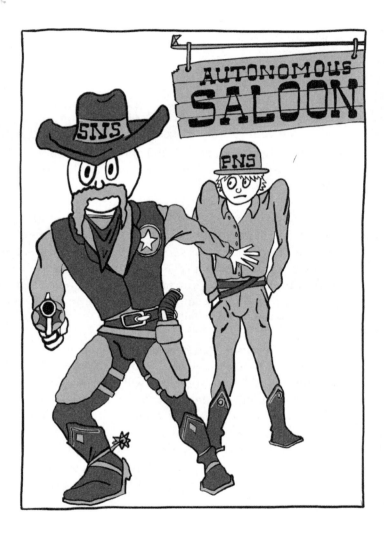

When the sympathetic nervous system is activated it will inhibit the parasympathetic nervous system.

Posture: Having a nice open posture, especially when sitting, is key to healthy diaphragmatic breathing. Avoid hunching over too much or leaning over to one side, leaning on your favourite arm. There are lots of expensive chairs out there but most chiropractors I know just use a blow-up exercise ball. We'll come back to posture in a bit more detail later on.

Time: Making time to do this simple exercise. It will only work if you do it. Far too many of my clients come to me because they are too busy and need to slow down, but then can't take five minutes to do these critical - even life-saving exercises.

We always have the time, we just need to prioritise these exercises and incorporate these changes into our daily lives. If we just focus on thinking of them as 'something else we need to do', we'll never start anything new…

(If you particularly struggle with this, an excellent read is *Atomic Habits* by James Clear. You won't look back.)

Consistency: Creating a routine or including introspective breathwork into your routine is key to success. I recommend performing your breathwork routine first and last thing in the day and, if you can, mid-morning and mid-afternoon. I've found these to be the most basic and effective times for a successful practice. These sessions can be just for a minute or two if that's all you've got, or for as long as it feels good.

Acute vs Chronic Stress
Though it may be more extreme in impact, acute stress is not only preferable to prolonged periods of lower level stress, otherwise known as chronic stress, but it has been demonstrated to be important for day-to-day growth and health.

Before we demonise chronic and worship acute stress let's break them down into what they are, and why each is bad or can be good for us.

We have already looked at what happens when the stress cycle kicks in. I hope we can agree that it is a beneficial process that has historically helped us to evolve into the complex being we see in the mirror every day.

We interpret danger, the stress cycle kicks in, we deal with the situation, flight/fight/freeze - and then the danger passes by. We live to fight another day or we've been eaten, either way it's the end of the equation.

However, as we've seen, the world we have created for ourselves has moved or evolved faster than we have been able to. This means our stress cycle is often not fit for purpose.

Instead we see danger everywhere. The stress-cycle constantly kicks in, we are unable to utilise it properly and so it keeps going like an old smokey generator in the back-room until it runs out of fuel. Then we crash.

Stress Breathing and an 'Acidic Body'

There's a lot of talk about acidification and alkalinity of the body in the wellness sector and, like everything, there are many facets to this and many false prophets too. Let's break it down so that it's super simple and you can start doing something about it right now.

The trigger to breathe in the body is caused by rising levels of carbon dioxide in the blood and not by falling oxygen levels. Our chemo-receptors that pick this-up actually detect for blood pH. Normal pH levels are between 7.35 and 7.45 and any variation in this will set off a chain of reactions.

When we are stressed we breathe more frequently and our blood-oxygen saturation percentage normally runs steadily in the high 90s. We can't take on all that much more oxygen, but when we over breathe (or hyperventilate) we dump carbon dioxide in quite dramatic levels. This can lead to our blood becoming too alkaline.

Turning back to the bus analogy, this means that if we breathe out too much carbon dioxide a strange thing happens. There are no carbon dioxide molecules left at the bus stop to hail the driver to stop, so they can swap seats with the oxygen molecules. The bus keeps on rolling along.

As we remain stressed throughout the day, sometimes right up to and including when we go to bed, this process continues. The buses keep running. They are packed full of oxygen wanting to go to work, but instead they pass by the factory gates looking forlornly out of the window at our industry base, as it remain empty and falls into disrepair.

Without the outgoing carbon dioxide molecules the oxygen can't get delivered to where it is needed most.

Without oxygen being delivered to our cells, they are deprived of energy, the acidity in our body has dropped, or has become *too* alkaline and this means that the bonding of the red blood cells to the oxygen molecules is strengthened. Our cells are therefore deprived of this essential component of life. As such we may start to interpret this as fatigue, aches and pains, which then eventually leads to cell death.

The causes can come from many causes, including heavy drug use to having had a stroke, but if we continue breathing this poorly for a long period of time, over the years, then our learned breathing pattern becomes too passive and too light to take in the oxygen we need in our body. At this stage things really aren't working correctly anymore, and carbon dioxide starts to build-up in our body and our blood. It is simply unable to be carried away simply because not longer enough buses are coming their way.

This build up of carbon dioxide causes an acidification (respiratory acidosis) which in turn causes it's own smorgasbord of problems, from diminishing bone density (as we literally dissolve our bones to balance the pH levels in our blood) to fatigue and a lack of sleep.

Whether our blood is alkaline or acidic, this is a concern for our general health and longevity of life. We want our blood to remain within the normal pH values to ensure all our bodily systems remain in sync.

Again we have good news, by practising breathwork techniques similar to 'Old Faithful' (the three-step breath process mentioned earlier) you will be able to balance out the carbon dioxide levels in your body, bit by bit until you are in complete harmony, floating in perfect homeostasis and feeling the blissful sunshine of equilibrium shining on your face.

There are of course many other exercises you can do, and nice progressions you can work on, but I'll list some of these at the end of the book. The urge to skip ahead may be huge but resist it if you can. Not only will you miss out on all my wonderful stories, but like most things in life, if you rush it, you'll only get some of the benefits. Breathwork takes time and the first big step is feeling into your breath and noticing what's really going on.

Panic Attacks
Just like my childhood doctor, there is a great deal of misunderstanding around panic attacks and breathing. I have been on a few workplace 'first aid' seminars where they recommend taking a few 'nice big deep breaths'. This is absolutely the wrong thing to do for a number of reasons.

First off, when you have got to the panic attack phase you are no longer in control of your breath - this is one of the definitions of a panic attack.

Secondly, over-breathing has caused/contributed the highly elevated stress levels and taking more deep breaths would simply extend your problems.

So, what's the answer - well, we don't need to look too far, in fact we can look to the traditional and low-tech solutions for the best results. Who remembers seeing people breathing into paper bags in comics and old movies? This is what we want to be doing.

We need to balance out the CO_2/O_2 in our bodies. We have breathed *out* all our CO_2, so that no matter how fast we are breathing we are no longer delivering the essential O_2 to our cells. Breathing in and out of a paper bag means we are *rebreathing* the CO_2 and slowly build back up our natural levels again. This then decreases the feeling of impending doom and the panic attack dissipates.

What if we don't have a paper bag. Despite environmental movements increasing the availability of paper over plastic bags in our immediate confines, we can improvise. Just cupping our hands together to form a chamber will lead to sufficient rebreathing of CO_2 to bring things back to normal. The health care professionals mean well, but a 'nice deep breath' is *not* always the answer to our problems.

NOTE: If by the end of this book, you are seriously concerned about your health and your stress levels, if you've tried the exercises listed in the text and you're still struggling to recover your natural breath then I'd recommend finding a local professional near you. If you go online you'll be able to find a trained functional breathwork coach near you (or online) - and with a similar mindset or background to yourself.

Chapter 6
Digestion

When we think about our health we often think of two main pillars. We think about our diet and exercise.

'A body is made in the kitchen and not the gym/made in the gym, revealed in the kitchen etc etc etc....'

Even a quick scan of the health and fitness industry, demonstrates that this makes-up the vast majority of articles, accounts and 'content'. Though there's no clear-cut definitive answers, it's worth remembering that everyone has an angle, especially those marketing themselves as influencers, they are however, all omitting a key factor.

Neither digestion nor exercise are possible without breathing. Both processes can be hindered by inefficient or dysfunctional breathing just as they can be maximised if a healthy breathing practice/healthy daily breathing is not in place.

Put very simply:

Food + Oxygen = Energy

Without food we can still get energy from burning through our fat reserves and metabolising muscle proteins, but without breath (or an efficient breath) we soon tire, cramp and then collapse.

If we were to test this using a little experiment, we could skip eating for a day and see how well we performed certain tasks. If, on the other hand, we were to skip breathing for a day, all our problem-solving days would be behind us… permanently.

We can keep going without food for a *lot* longer than we can without a breath, we don't need to experiment on each-other to know this. Our breath is more immediately important than a snack.

If we remember back to why we breathe, and how the oxygen combines with glucose to create ATP (adenosine triphosphate) aka *energy*, this then allows movement, thought and heat generation as well as giving off water and carbon dioxide.

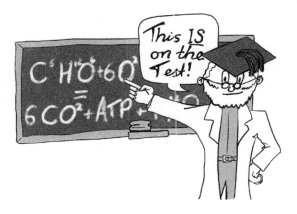

Without effective or efficient oxygen delivery we won't be able to metabolise energy in the cells. If we are breathing poorly, whether it's over breathing caused by excessive stress or by physiological problems such as mouth-breathing, we starve our cells of the vital energy they need. We touched on the dangers of chronic stress, and its effect on illness and injury in the previous chapters, but let's back it up a step and go really basic and proper old school.

As we have already seen, the autonomic nervous system is split into two components. There is the sympathetic and the parasympathetic. We've had a look at their roles already but let's think about the common names they have been given:

'Fight and Flight'
and
'Rest and Digest'

These are often thought of as mutually exclusive. You can be in one state or another. This is of course an oversimplification but it's generally the case. I like to think of it like a see-saw (teeter-totter for my American friends). As one goes up so the other conversely comes down, or as one is stimulated, so the other is suppressed.

When we are constantly in a stressed or over stressed state then we cannot by definition go into the 'rest and digest 'phase. Blood flow is restricted from our gut by the constant release of cortisol. This means that optimum blood-flow to our guts, to help the breakdown and harvest of nutrients, is restricted. We are unable to fulfil this simple and necessary function.

As healthily as we may be eating, if we are over-breathing, if we are in a frequently stressed state of being, then we simply won't be able to make the most of the nutrients and energy in the food we eat.

This is another one of those 'Eureka! 'moments - but it's also something that most of us already knew. Simply saying it aloud it becomes kind of blindingly obvious. All we had to do was stop and think about it, again something that we're simply not encouraged to do.

The fact that healthy breathing is not featured as one of the pillars of healthy living is beyond me. It should be right up there with diet and exercise; the perfect three-legged stool of health and fitness. Actually, let's throw away the three-legged stool. Everyone always analogies about these, let's use an old fashioned chair. We need diet, healthy breathing, exercise and rest/recovery for healthy living and/or to get fit.

Breathing normally with slow, deep breaths through the nose, and using the diaphragm will allow us to balance our autonomic nervous system as much as possible. We give the digestion of food the space and energy it needs. Digestion is a lengthy process. In a healthy body, it takes around three days from eating to pooping (unless it's sweetcorn...). We need to create a safe and stress-free space for our body to break down the food we eat. For healthy digestion, think candles and classical music rather than strobe lights and techno.

In the wild, we would have generally experienced higher states of stress for short moments in an average day. Now we are in a constant flux, often from when we wake to when we try and go to sleep. Messing-up our digestion is just another aspect of this unhealthy process that will lead us towards fatigue, illness, and eventually an earlier death.

So, we can either try and squeeze in extreme moments of calm, we can 'meditate the shit 'out of ourselves in the mornings, we can rush to a yoga or breathwork class to balance us back out again - or we can try and breathe more steadily throughout the day, bringing more balance and stability into our everyday. Or, we can do all of the above.

Cell Metabolism and Fatigue

When I suffered from stress and anxiety 24:7 I was alway tired. I had to drag myself out of bed in the morning, I mainlined coffee and tea, often washing-down sugary snacks all day long just to keep going. Then, come evening time I'd drink a few beers or a bottle of wine and try to shut-down my racing (though erratic) mind. Often I'd also use sleeping tablets ranging from valerian to codeine.

Then the next day, after an erratic and too short a night's sleep I'd go at it all over again. Too many of us find ourselves in this downward spiral and wish-away our lives until the weekend or the next holiday, where we can collapse on a lounger by the pool and drink an oversized cocktail at lunchtime.

When we are stressed, we operate on adrenaline and fumes alone. I was certainly addicted to this lifestyle - since starting as a chef in my early twenties I was a fully fledged, card-carrying member of the 'Burn the Candle at Both Ends! 'club and drove myself steadily and rapidly towards the cliff edge. Luckily for me, when I eventually fell over the edge I landed on another ledge. Many of us aren't so lucky.

Fortunately for me I hit burn-out and had a mental breakdown before my body shut down completely and I died. Without over-dramatising it, I came close a few times.

As well as our own we can learn from others 'mistakes - we can recognise behavioural patterns in our own lives and hopefully start to make some informed decisions *before* we get to breaking point.

When we are stressed we activate the sympathetic nervous system - we go into fight or flight whether this is what we actually *need* or not. This suppresses our parasympathetic nervous system - our rest and digest and, well... the results are blindingly obvious now we can see them, we cannot rest and we cannot digest.

This sends our body into overdrive - as if we are firing a nitro-boost into an empty fuel tank.

We keep blood and energy away from our digestion process and we over-breathe, meaning that we cannot get the oxygen to the cells in our body and the parts of the brain that we need. The effect is equivalent to not putting any wood onto the fire and starving it of oxygen, meaning the fire just sputters out.

This is one of the few bodily functions I struggled to understand. For the most part our body behaves in the right way in most given situations. We have an in-built survival instinct. The answer is, of course, simple once light is shone on the issue, and we have already covered it a few times. It is because we have taken ourselves out of our natural surroundings. When we are stressed we press that Big Red Button and breathe even faster. We keep this up, doing untold damage to ourselves and only stop in extreme circumstances when our body says 'ENOUGH' and hits the 'reset 'button and we pass-out, or faint. Then our breathing returns to normal again.

Without either oxygen or glucose delivery we starve our cells of basic energy, we starve our bodies of life itself.

It's no wonder we feel so damn tired!

The Cult of Busy

So we find ourselves depleted of energy, we cannot focus or concentrate, our temper is on a hair-trigger and, to put it simply, we feel like shit.

As far as our body and its struggle to survive these hostile conditions goes - it's just plain flummoxed. We wouldn't *deliberately* be putting ourselves in this extreme and continued state of stress and damage would we? Of course not. So, as if we had been plonked in the middle of the Sahara with no water, our body fires on all pistons/full-speed ahead, until we are out of danger.

Except this is our daily life.

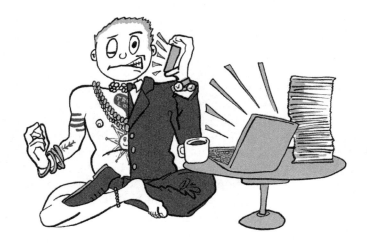

This is how we live and spend most of our days, weeks and years in this modern world we have created for ourselves… This is the grind which we not only accept but embrace and celebrate.

Our modern Cult of Being Busy ('I'll sleep when I'm dead) celebrates the sacrifices we make to the altar of work. We applaud self-destruction in the name of success and later on laugh at horror stories over a shared beer, or ten. We keep pushing to the breaking point where we either collapse, are overtaken or replaced or we make it limping to our holiday where we finally get to stop - and stop we do - normally by getting ill immediately and spending a few days in bed, unable to enjoy the short amount of leisure time we have in the sun.

So, how does our body keep going? Emergency signals are being sent out with such regularity that we seek stimulants when the adrenaline is depleted. I never did it myself but most chefs I knew lived on cocaine. This was just to get through the day, not as a party drug in the evening - well, often both to be fair, but mostly just to get through the day.This isn't just found in professional kitchens of old, it's common practice in many places of work from PR offices to politics, banking to customer service: all of these toxic workplaces that put output ahead of wellbeing and drive us to these self-destructive behaviours.

Binge Eating

This all means that no matter how carefully or well we eat, we're not getting the nutrients and energy from food. We aren't getting the requisite oxygen delivered to the cells, so we aren't getting the energy through the air we breathe. We go into a sort of free-fall and emergency setting.

Signals are sent via the sympathetic nervous system to breathe faster as 'we need more air 'but we've seen how this paradox works. Breathing faster just means less oxygen delivered to the cells that need it the most. It starves them.

So we seek a quick fix for energy NOW! We need to bypass our defunctive (suppressed) digestion system and we need that boost before we come to a complete stand still. 'Luckily 'for us with our modern food systems and supermarkets, we have all this rocket-fuel close at hand.

And so we start to crave, seek and devour sugary and fatty foods even more than normal. We need energy and as pure sugar is readily available and close at hand, we plug it into our veins, open the valve and let it flow on in!

When we think of someone who is chronically stressed we picture a thin, twitchy individual with nicotine-stained fingers, coffee breath and a very poor complexion. But as we find ourselves drifting towards this ideal, instead of cutting back on what we know isn't doing us any good, we continue reaching for these quick fixes and add in all the masking tools too: mouthwash, moisturisers, make-up, nice clothes and a fresh hairdo.

We can also find ourselves stress-eating. This is a very real and very dangerous addiction. At least we are eating and not letting our body cannibalise itself from within but this is still no way to live, and it only brings another raft of health and psychological issues into play as we drift down the river of life.

We are stressed and over-breathing, we have an acidic system and on top of this, we are consuming refined and processed sugar in whatever form we can find. From biscuits to beer, Haribos become our new heroin as we chase that sugar high.

Along with caffeine and maybe cigarettes and cocaine too, these soon become the only things keeping us going.

In the words of Anchorman Ron Burgundy:

'Boy, that escalated quickly!'

So, let's take a little break to take a breath…

Through no fault of our own we find ourselves overstressed and out of control. We lose the ability to breathe healthily and shove sugar and stimulants into our bodies with abandon.

This is no real way to live. We have the tools and knowledge to break that chain. By focusing on our breath and introducing healthier breathing habits we can 'take back control '(but in a healthy and non-Brexity kind of way).

Through learning to breathe healthily, and bringing these

principles into our daily lives, we are able to not only break this self-destructive chain but we are also able to reverse the damage already done.

Additional benefits that will come our way are: increased concentration, better moods, a reduction of brain-fog, weight management and better sleep, to mention a few.

Chapter 7
Stress and our Immune System

It's generally understood that the higher and more continuous our stress levels are, the poorer health we have. When we feel stressed and burnt-out we seem to catch every cold that's going around, have more sick days at work and our mood suffers greatly, even nudging us into a depressed state. Let's take a step back and look at the complex interplay that stress has specifically on our immune system, and how the way we breathe affects both.

Just like with our digestive system, when our fight and flight mode is engaged we suppress our immediate immune system, as our body's priority is in getting out of danger and not so much fighting a cold we may have picked-up. Problems really start to escalate though, when we are continuously in our fight or flight, or when it fires so often our body never recovers in between bouts and so never returns to 'normal'.

We have already established the direct relationship that our breathing has on our stress levels and conversely the effect that stress has on our breathing patterns, let's take a closer look and see how that plays out with all three levels of our immune system.

Our Immune System
A brief overview of the systems that have evolved in humans to keep us healthy are split into three levels, some we share with plants and bacteria and others are unique to mammals who eat

with a mouth. For these reasons we evolved to have three immune systems in operation. These consist of the primary, the innate and the adaptive immune systems, but rather than think of them as three independent processes, we can look at it like three waves of defence in our overall immune system.

Primary Defence

The first barrier against any infection or pathogens getting into our body is our skin. This literal wall is made of three parts, the epidermis, dermis and subcutaneous (fatty) layers. Cuts, grazes and maimings aside, this barrier effectively stops anything harmful in the surrounding environment from getting into our bodies and causing us problems.

On average we have nine holes or openings into our bodies (from mouth to genitals). These are the only natural breaks in this physical barrier. At each of these sites for possible incursion we have developed different tactics to repel foreign invaders.

Focussing on breathing, let's look at the mouth and nose.

First off we have some mechanical defences. Coughing and sneezing might not be pleasant for those around us, and many illnesses have co-opted this for their own ability to spread and grow, but generally these act as a good way to forcibly expel many harmful particulates.

If harmful particulates or bacteria get past this line of defence, then our nose has a few things up its proverbial sleeve. Our nose hairs and cilia act as sticky traps and our mucus membranes can soon be brought into action to help catch, hold and transport problem intruders down into the fiery pit of hell that is our stomach. In addition to this process is the chemical weapon of nitric oxide - our old friend and Nobel Prize winner - which is also a powerful antibacterial agent.

If we happen to be breathing through our mouth a lot, or all of the time, we may catch some intruding microorganisms in mucus in our throat but apart from this we are leaving ourselves open for attack. Yet again, the best line of defence we have is to breathe through our nose.

Inflammation in the body

Our innate immune system is, as the name suggests, something that we are born with. Passed down through our hereditary lines, this complex array of white blood cells and their supporting teams locate and attack pathogens, once they have broken through the primary lines of defence. Our most common experience of this, is when we get an infected cut, graze or sting. The active agents rush to the scene of the incursion and signalling agents (cytokines and interleukins) point to where attention is needed and red and white blood cells rush in, causing swelling to occur.

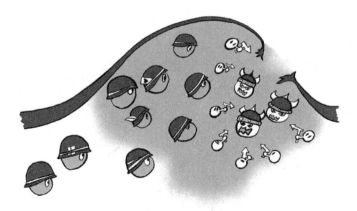

White blood cells identify and attack foreign bodies

Inflammation is a common and effective component of our innate immune system. As all hands are on deck, our body responds effectively, if sometimes over-zealously to foreign cells, be they bacteria, viruses, cancers or even organ transplants. This results in swelling which can be red, sore and hot and this is due to this fervent activity just below (and inside) our skin. Platelets in our blood block any cuts, to both stop any blood loss but also to stop any further infection. White blood cells either lock onto alien invaders/antigens or they start to consume them altogether. As simple as this may sound this is an incredibly complex process.

In normal stress and sleep cycles, cortisol is known to reduce our inflammatory response. We release higher levels during waking hours, and this naturally inhibits swelling and energy being directed to healing during the lighter hours of the day. Remembering that we are animals, we need to be out searching for food, strengthening social bonds and generally doing our thing during the day. When we are lying still at night this is the perfect time for the body to heal and repair itself and it is one of the reasons sleep is so important. If we disrupt our sleeping pattern too regularly we face breaking our natural healing rhythms.

However, due to our non-animalistic lifestyles and our disconnect from natural rhythms, our cortisol levels are higher than desired and when we find ourselves in a chronic state of stress, our adaptive immune system gets knocked completely out of sync. It's not entirely known why this is, but it is yet another victim of modern life. The further we stray from our bodies balance, from homeostasis, the less well our bodily systems seem to behave.

In the case of inflammation in the body it becomes self-destructive, cytokines which normally have a 'task and finish ' role start to over-react, and are produced in larger numbers, hang around past their welcome and cause excessive swelling.

This all exacerbates or even creates inflammatory problems, causing a plethora of health issues from arthritis to arteriosclerosis and from depression to cancer.

Adaptive Immune System

Unlike many aspects of the medical world, our immune system is named in 'plain english'. As the name suggests, the adaptive immune system functions at a higher level: it adapts to meet new threats and pathogens. Depending on the environment we are in, we learn from past infections so that the next time we are threatened, our body is immediately suited to fight it off.

We create an 'immunological memory': our long life white blood cells (WBC) recognises the threat using a signature antigen. After the first initial attack, our defensive forces are issued with a permanent ID of alien invaders. Apologies for any over-use of military-style terminology here but the parallels are just too close.

And so here we go, our troops are the lymphocytes - two types T and B Cells (originating from the thyroid or bone marrow respectively) B cells identify, tag and signal. Killer T cells are on a specific search and destroy mission, killing host cells that are infected to stop the spread of any infection. Helper T cells assist the process by directing the attacking white blood cells to their specific role or target.

Unlike with the innate immune system, it seems our adaptive system comes into its own during waking hours and rests at night. Considering our animal (and human) status, we are more likely to be coming into contact with new and strange pathogens during our waking hours than we are when fast asleep in our 'cave'. As such, concentrations of T lymphocytes and natural killer cells peak at much higher levels during the daytime.

Natural killer cells play an essential role in weeding out and destroying damaging growths in the body, including tumours and cancers. Their role has been demonstrated to be affected and limited by chronic stress. While there is a lot of controversy around stress, and the causation and worsening of cancer in the scientific community, it is agreed that a high stress lifestyle both increases our chances of developing cancer in the first place and that once established, it will compound its spread.

The exact causation links between stress and its effect on the innate and adaptive immune system, are still not entirely known, but this is an area of research and concern and the more that is discovered, the clearer the causation link is. In the meantime, it *is* known that our breathing patterns and exercises, we can use, do reduce stress and this has had the positive effect of preventing and reducing inflammation in the body and the resulting illness associated with it.

Breathing on Prescription
Though many health professionals now suggest relaxation and health-positive activities, from yoga to deep breathwork, such activities are still not available on most public health plans. In a recent interview with Denise Shipani, Alka Gupto, MD and co-director of integrated heath at The Brain and Spine Institute at Weill Cornell Medicine in New York said:

'We do know, though, that when we teach people how to reduce stress in whatever form - stress management tips, classes, individual advice, yoga, deep breathing - we see decreases in some of these inflammatory side effects.'

Our breath can and does affect our health, and, just as with stress, this can be a positive or negative feedback loop. The choice is ours with every breath we take.

The connection is now clear between our respiratory system, nervous system and immune system. We know that healthy, efficient diaphragmatic nasal breathing is the foundation of a healthy life. We filter out and destroy most pathogens, ensure our sleep cycles (and therefore our rest and repair processes) operate properly and we enable a perfect battle field for our white blood cells to fight any infections, incursions and abnormal growths.

In addition to this, recent discoveries around forced and conscious over-breathing suggests we can directly strengthen our immune systems by the way we breathe. Deliberately over-breathing, and incorporating breath-holds, creates a temporary hypoxic and hypo/hypercapnia state (low oxygen in the body and low/high carbon dioxide levels in the blood). This seems to recreate the rare, high stress situations we'd find ourselves in living as animals in the wild. We then put the control of the immune system back into the hands of the breather.

Built on ancient Pranayama and Tummo practices, modern breathing celebrities such as Wim Hof (copyright) have famously championed these and other powerful breathing techniques. Though similar in effect to hyperventilation such techniques differ drastically as it is only for a short and specific time period and it is the breather who is fully in control.

Scientific research into' The Wim Hof Method / WHM'(copyright) has demonstrated that the innate immune system can be temporarily subdued through the conscious triggering of eustress in the body, and that breath-holds stimulate new blood production and bolster the adaptive immune system too.

Whatever method we use, when we deliberately hold our breath for continuous periods of time, our blood oxygen drops to 'unnatural 'levels. If done frequently, we send an emergency signal to our bone marrow to create more blood. This is just one of the natural processes that can be 'hacked 'for our benefit. When our body makes new red blood cells, we automatically also build new white blood cells too.

NOTE: Any strong breathwork and breath-hold practice should only ever be performed and learned under the eye of a professional breathwork practitioner who is specifically trained in the practice and has proper first aid knowledge, insurance and certification.

Chapter 8
Sleep

As an ex-insomniac who still sometimes suffers from a lack of sleep, it would be remiss of me not to include a section on sleep. Sleep really is another cornerstone of our general health, and not getting enough can have severe short and long term effects.

For decades I'd never get a good night's sleep. My high adrenaline/high stress lifestyle meant that I was always on the go, and combined with my generally overanxious nature it was near impossible to 'switch-off' in the evenings when my head hit the pillow.

This formed who I was and also my mental image of myself. In my mind's eye, I was a 'deep-thinker', a night owl and, because the collapse was yet to come, I was someone who didn't need sleep. These were the days before social media but we were still aware of famous and successful people who got by on just a few hours sleep a night. With the rose-tinted glasses of my early twenties, I was destined for fame, fortune and greatness and sleep wasn't going to get in my way!

Now, with the gift of hindsight and hundreds of hours of reflective conscious breathwork, I'm able to peel away the layers and see it for what it was. I was an overworked, underpaid chef who had a mildly healthy delusion of grandeur. My high stress job and mouth-breathing had knocked my hormonal systems out of whack and I was getting by on cortisol and coffee alone.

I'd stay out late and developed an aversion to sleep. I believed it was my enemy. Lack of sleep served to further cloud my judgement so I ended-up convinced these self-destructive habits were good for me in the long run. When my drunk head would eventually hit the pillow, it was because I was about to collapse anyway and I'd pass out. This was low quality and in no way restorative sleep and for not nearly enough time.

But *everyone* was tired in the mornings - we were night owls! We just had to get it together enough to get through the day. We'd mainline stimulants (personally avoiding the cocaine that was everywhere) and by around ten in the morning we'd start to feel OK again, and start laughing about the crazy nights we'd had and the painful mornings-after.

This was back in the day before I started getting hangovers. This was a super-power I must have been genetically blessed with, or perhaps cursed with, as I kept drinking unhealthy amounts well into my forties to help unwind in the evenings, but that's a whole other book.

I'd almost trained myself to not need sleep. As with many dysfunctional behaviours, this worked out 'just fine', until it didn't.

As I nudged into my thirties I'd need to wake in the night for a pee, then more than once, and as my heartburn and chronic acid reflux got worse, this could keep me awake and staring red-eyed at the ceiling, listening to Bill Hicks CDs and Radio 4, desperately yearning for the respite of at least a few hours sleep. Finally, I'd start to drift off just before my alarm rang.

I'd try all the top tips, from black-out blinds to less spicy foods, but of course drinking less caffeine and alcohol was out of the question (these balanced each other out anyway right?). I tried to cut down on blue light before bed, but by this stage I was so busy working and emailing right up to the point when I went to bed, that this just wasn't realistic. I also tried everything else, including sleeping pills.

This was not long before my first collapse and breakdown.

There are now many readily-available top tips that we can employ to help us to get a better night's sleep and here's a list below, adapted from the 'health-line 'website. But until we address the issue of our breathing, we'll never tackle the root of the problem:

- Increase natural light during the day and reduce and cut blue light exposure for two hours before bed
- Reduce your caffeine intake and stop drinking alcohol
- Implement a regular sleeping routine, including any naps
- Consider using melatonin and other natural sleep-cycle supplements
- Optimise your bedroom. Create a comfy, quiet, cool and dark environment
- Don't eat before bed
- Take a relaxing bath or shower, relax clear your mind (including deep breathing) in the evenings

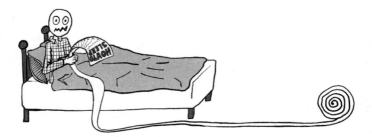

It is only at the very end of the list that breathing is brought into the equation, but healthy and deep breathing should be first and foremost as well as a central part of, not just our pre-sleep period, but our entire day itself.

Pre-Sleep

As we know, and my story at the start of this chapter demonstrated, a stressful lifestyle is not conducive to our health. As I did with everything in my twenties, I pushed everything to the extreme, but sadly it leached into my thirties and then forties too. When we are overly triggering our stress response and living in an almost constant state of 'fight or flight', our health suffers.

We've already looked at many elements of this, but a constant 'on 'setting for our sympathetic nervous system is going to have disastrous effects on our sleep. As sleep is generally regarded as the time the body rests, rebuilds, repairs and recharges itself, doing anything that hampers this process is an act of self-sabotage.

Dr Mark Burhenne, author of *The 8 Hour Sleep Paradox* recently reiterated that:

'Without quality sleep, NOTHING else matters.

You won't make the right decisions with diet and you won't have the energy or motivation to work out.

Make airway health your #1 priority.'

Our mind races, we are unable to 'turn-off '*because* we are in a sympathetic state from all the activities during the day. This then causes us frustration and anxiety and we keep this physiological and mental state going. We spiral into our insomnia, just as we spiral into our anxiety attack at work, until it gets so bad our internal dialogue becomes savage and cannibalistic.

But just as we can take control through our breathing during the day to stop rising anxiety, so we can do the same in the evening:

Breathing Exercise to Slow a Racing Mind

- Start by focusing on your breath.
- We aren't judging ourselves, we are simply observing our breath.
- Feel into the connection between our breath and how we feel, our emotional state, our racing heart and mind.
- There is no rush, be kind to yourself.
- This awareness is the first step. From here we will slowly start change where we breathe so that our breath is beginning in the belly, with the diaphragm.
- Then start to see if you can breath in through the nose alone.
- This may take some attempts but go slowly and remain judgement free.
- Finally start to focus on your breaths and count as you do so, in for four, out for five, pause for a second and then repeat.
- Gradually start exhaling for longer and let your in-breath become even more gentle and lighter.
- Repeat until you sleep.

Starting Early

Long before you are ready for bed, and after your evening meal, start to match your breaths to your activity.

Unless you are exercising try and focus on nice light but deep breaths. In through the nose and deep into your belly, and again we can follow the in for four, out for five, rest and repeat pattern, but simple light and deep breaths is enough.

This is a perfect exercise to do while sitting watching tv or a movie, your posture needn't be perfect as long as you are comfortable.

This helps us double-fold by enabling us to both realise when it's time for bed and then helping us transition beautifully from day into night - and sleep.

The Military Method

This is a popular method that's been doing the circuits online for a few years now. Those serving in the armed forces are often under high stress, and their bodies need to recover more than average. It combines both breathing methods, tension release and visualisation.

You can also download a nice yoga nidra app (they say these aren't for sleep but I've found them to be excellent).

- Relax your jaw and face muscles. Let your tongue loll in your mouth.
- Drop your shoulders down, letting go of any held tension.
- Let your arms sit loose by your sides, and relax your hands and fingers.
- Exhale deeply and relax your chest, then feel that relaxation flow down through your body to your legs and feet.
- Imagine a warm, calming sensation flowing from your head to your feet.
- Inhale and exhale letting your mind clear and if thoughts pop-up say: 'Don't think, don't think 'ten times.
- Now visualise yourself in a hammock in the pitch black or lying in a canoe beneath a beautiful night sky.
- See you in the morning.

During Sleep

When we suffer from sleep problems and disorders, we may wake at many points during the night. This can be from a number of causes from mouth breathing - raising our stress levels, causing our mind to race and anxiety to creep into our sanctuary of sleep, through to our need to pee.

Antidiuretic hormone (ADH) is normally released during deep sleep and inhibits our need to pee. Needing to urinate is generally a sign that we have entered into a very light sleep, rather than our needing to pee has woken us up. ADH stops being released and we need to trudge to the loo. It can of course be a sign of urinary tract infection or other problems but mostly it's caused by light sleeping.

If we've been drinking alcohol, which is a diuretic, then expect the bladder to be full and the floodgates to be opened multiple times a night.

Waking multiple times during the night disrupts our sleep rhythm and often means we are unable to get into the really beneficial deep-sleep states/brain waves, where our body repairs and recovers after a hard day. If we wake and don't need the loo, or if we do and struggle to fall-asleep again, any of the exercises listed above will help. Most importantly of all though, make sure you start nasal breathing straight away, even (or especially) if you need to put on slippers and go down flights of stairs or along a corridor to the toilet.

If we keep waking with a start, snore loudly or simply keep waking multiple times a night, this could be a sign of sleep-apnea and it is best to catch this as early as possible. All the advice contained here can and will help, but it is advisable to also seek out a doctors assessment.

Mouth Tape

This practice is still often seen as quite a drastic intervention, despite its recent rise in popularity. Mouth taping can be seen as a really intrusive, extreme and drastic measure but the opposite is the case. When used correctly, mouth taping is so safe that it can be used with children to help create safe and healthy sleep patterns. It's a simple way to nudge us into breathing through our nose while sleeping.

My mum tried everything to help me sleep better, and had we known about this practice when I was a kid, it's safe to say we could have cracked my insomnia at an early age and a whole plethora of problems could have been averted. But then I was also a bit of a 'turd' when it came to bedtime (my words not my mum's). My refusal to go to sleep was so strong, that apparently sometimes I'd be softly snoring with eyes wide open.

Mouth-taping has also gotten a bad rep by some influencers recently. They are those people, bad apples made worse on the internet. Their aims are to get hits and likes instead of passing on helpful advice and in doing so, they always seem to take things too far. N*ever* use duct-tape. *Never* completely cover your whole mouth and *never*, and I mean *NEVER-EVER...* tape the whole way around your head!

Rather than stopping us from breathing through our mouth, taping persuades us to breathe through our nose instead. This brings the whole raft of benefits we have already discussed around nasal breathing and helps us slip into, and stay in, a nice deep and restorative night's sleep.

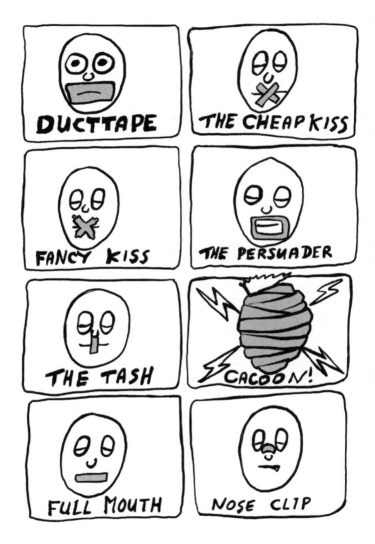

To mouth-tape on not-to mouth-tape,
that is not the only question…

How to Mouth Tape

It is very simple to apply. We simply want to hold or persuade the lips together, but while maintaining gaps so that any urgent breaths, sneezes or coughs can still escape without a barrier. Two excellent ways are to place a thin strip of tape in the centre of our mouth so the edges are clear, or use a special tape that goes around the outside and nudges the lips together.

After brushing and flossing our teeth, and before we turn off the light, is a good time to apply it, depending on what other evening activities you have planned, or that happen unplanned. If for any reason the tape comes loose or comes unstuck, we can simply reapply it or replace it with a new strip. For this reason, I'd recommend keeping some beside the bed and popping it on as you are thinking about going to sleep.

I have a beard, and this sometimes restricts my ability to get full purchase but as we use it more, the less tape we actually need for it to be effective. Now my sleeping patterns and behaviours have improved, I only really use it when needed, but many people I know still use it every night regardless.

What tape to buy

As the practice has increased in popularity, there are now many products we can choose from. I now use cheap and readily available medical tape for about 50p a roll. We want to use the surgical tape that is sticky but in *no* way sticks so much that it damages the delicate skin around our lips when we peel it off. You can go with well known brands such as 3M, or any 'own brand' that your local chemist offers.

You can buy specially made X shaped gel tapes to go over the mouth but, a little 2cm strip in the middle of the mouth performs the same purpose. If you want a cute X shape then you can do this with the surgical tape too.

Another great solution is the Buteyko brand of tape that sits around the outside of the lips and gently holds them together. This may look and feel a bit strange at first, and isn't great if you have a beard, but it's excellent as an introductory method and to get into the practice. You also soon realise that a good night's sleep outweighs any concerns you may have about how you look while sleeping. Besides, trust me, your partner will have seen and heard a lot worse!

Essentially, as with anything though - whatever works best for you is the way to go. Try a few different types of tape and techniques, and go with what works best for you. We are all different and this is what makes the world such an exciting and wonderful place!

JUST DON'T USE DUCT TAPE.

Post Sleep / All Day

We now understand the relationship between our breathing and the arousal/stress cycle. We've seen how our breathing can affect our stress levels and vice-versa. Most importantly, we know how our breathing can help us to break this cycle, and install a healthy and sustaining one in its place.

One of the most important things we can do to ensure a good night's sleep, is to ensure we breathe better during the day. Rather than put more pressure on ourselves at this stage, with the knowledge we now have, this is simply what we are all doing or striving to do now anyway, and we'll reap the benefits together.

A healthy breathing practice during the day will contribute towards a healthy breathing practice at night. Conversely, how we breathe at night affects how well we sleep. This then affects how well we rest and recover and therefore how well we will breathe the following day. Just as a stressful breath will trigger a stressful feeling, so will a stressful day of breathing trigger a stressful nights sleep - or lack thereof - and we can just as easily flip this on it's head and create a healthy and nurturing practice in its place.

Maintaining a healthy breathing pattern while at work and play during the day, will mean less of a drastic need to shift into 'sleep mode 'come nighttime. We won't need to take such urgent action or spend ages doing specific exercises, trying as hard as we can to relax in the first place. We'll simply transition into that natural next phase of our day and drift into luxurious and delightful sleep...

Performing breathing exercises, maintaining an open posture and staying away from too many stimulants during the day, will allow us to manage stress better when it arrives. If we have also been practising exercises to increase our tolerance to carbon dioxide, we will likewise be able to manage our response to stress when it enters our lives. Breathing through our nose, and ensuring our diaphragm is used in every breath, we'll maintain balance and pose, again more sure-footed in our defence against the harmful effects of stress.

This all helps us sleep better later on.

Sports Performance and Recovery

As we have seen, sports performance will improve the better our breathing becomes. From more efficient digestion to better energy, breathing better will help our performance better on and off the pitch. Combined with the CO2 paradox which we'll address soon we start to become turbo-charged, but let's also look at the essential role of sleep.

During sleep our body focuses on *rest and repair*. Our energy goes into repairing damaged cells, fighting any possible invaders and building new ones. If we are physically active it's likely we will injure or tear our muscles. In fact, for our muscles to grow we actively *need* to micro-tear them. Sleep is the time we grow and also when we recover.

As such it is an essential part of any athlete's training programme whether they are an olympic weight lifter or a Saturday morning footballer. Sleep is a critical part of our health and growth and more so for athletes.

Eustress is Good Stress

Embracing a form of eustress (deliberate exposure to a high stress for a short amount of time) can also be hugely beneficial in balancing out our stressful lives. It's almost mimicking the bursts we'd have experienced living in the wild.

Forms of eustress can vary and be anything from a nice HIIT (high intensity interval training) session in the gym to jumping in a cold showers. Some people need to bungee jump or skydive, but incorporating these short sharp shock treatments helps us flush out the artificial stress peaks in our daily grind. Whatever form this takes, finding something that works for you is massively beneficial, as long as it's in moderation. If we embrace this lifestyle *too much* then we'll overtax and endanger our systems to too much stress anyway.

I like to think of this process as a bit of a jet-wash for our autonomic nervous system, blasting away all the crap and leaving it nice and shiny at the end, back to our balance level or, as I say, our state of readiness, where we can be in charge of where our nervous system goes, ramping it up when needed and bringing it down when required. Putting ourselves in the driving seat, rather than the uncontrollable factors in our daily lives.

Combining a healthy breathing pattern during the day with controlled spikes due to activities we find fun but challenging, we are able to maintain a healthy balance and ensure we're best placed to drift into the evening and eventually a good night's sleep.

There's always a time when we'll need to firefight. When we find insomnia creeping in, there are exercises we can do to counteract the rising stress in our systems, but most important is the knowledge that we *are* in control and we can do something about it.

If you try these techniques and your sleeping disorders persist, if you snore at night, then seek professional sleep assessment and treatment. It may seem like an excessive step but so did mouth-tape once upon a time. A good night's sleep is important and we need to look after ourselves as well as we look after those that we love.

Chapter 9
The CO2 Paradox

(For the purpose of ease, as we'll be mentioning carbon dioxide / CO2 so many times in this chapter, we'll use the shortened term.)

There's a lot of misinformation and misunderstanding around one of life's essential gases. CO2 has gained a really bad rep recently and it's wholly unjustified. Last time I checked, CO2 wasn't wearing a black and white stripy top, breaking into people's homes, nor was he lighting fires and burning our planet's ancient stores of fossil fuels for shareholder profit.

CO2 isn't the 'bad-guy', he's just become confused with a lot of the really bad stuff that's going on right now. Sure, anthropological climate change is one of the biggest problems our generations can face and high levels of CO2 are responsible for the gradual warming of the planet, but this is a by-product of *our* actions and it's in no way the fault of our friend CO2. He's just going about his business helping to create the building blocks of life as he always has.

CO2 is what plants inhale, we learn this at school, it's a crucial part of the circle of life. Plants inhale CO2 and exhale O2, while we and other mammals inhale O2 and exhale CO2. It's almost as if it's perfect by design, but like most things in nature, it has taken a VERY long time indeed to find this perfect balance.

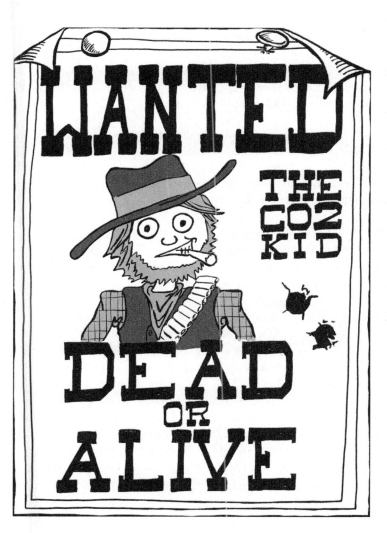

Carbon dioxide isn't the villain it's often made out to be

This inherent carbon then goes on to be the essential building blocks of almost every form of life we know of. So it's a pretty big deal, hats-off to Mr and Mrs CO2!

But that's not where the bum-rap for CO2 ends. We know that we breathe *out* CO2 and so it must be a waste product. Waste is 'bad' therefore CO2 must be 'bad' too.

On deeper inspection we also find that higher levels of CO2 in the blood and body means our body is in an acidic state. We know that an acidic body can lead to all kinds of health problems, in the short and long term. CO2 contributes to acidification, therefore it must be bad.

By this stage I couldn't help but think that if CO2 was a cowboy in the Wild West he would have already been chased down by our wayward hero of a bounty hunter and handed over to the authorities for a swift and very public execution.

However, just like many public executions, they would have got the wrong guy. CO2 is actually a friend of ours and, dropping the wild west metaphors for a while, it's an element that is essential for our health, performance and the existence of life itself.

Recent investigation into this has gained great momentum, and we are finally redefining the role and importance of CO2 in our day to day health, and continued strive for athletic excellence. If you want to learn more about this issue, check out the works of Patrick McKeown. His 'Oxygen Advantage 'programmes and work with the Buteyko Clinic, has pulled together and built on the scientific discoveries in this field. A lot of the information in this chapter is drawn from the excellent work in this field. So let's take a deeper look!

A By-product with Important Roles

CO_2 is indeed a by-product of our respiration. As we've already covered, when we breathe, we absorb O_2 through the permeable membranes in the alveoli - or air sacs - in our lungs. This O_2 is then transported to our cells, where it is used to create energy and life itself.

After this process, one of the byproducts is CO_2, as well as water, but we don't go demonising water (yet, just give the British press a few weeks…). This CO_2 is carried by our same blood, back to our same alveolus, into our same lungs and we exhale it out into the atmosphere for our happy plants to consume. And so it goes on.

But of course the process isn't quite as simple as all this. Finding a common ground of understanding, let's return to the bus analogy we have used previously and remind ourselves of the critical role that CO_2 has to play within our bodies, and how we can harness it to our advantage.

All Aboard!

It's all very well to just assume that the O_2 we breathe in is going to find its way into the cells that need it most, or in fact to all the cells in the body, but when we stop and think about this, it is a mammoth task. Our blood vessels alone can be stretched out to over 100,000km. They would travel around the world two and a half times! How do the fresh-faced little O_2 molecules know where to go, and where to leave the bloodstream?

Going back to the bus analogy I love so much - our blood is full of red blood cells (RBCs): these in turn have haemoglobin which are the bonds that allow them to carry oxygen throughout our body and then carry the CO_2 away again.

The RBCs have their briefcases packed and are ready to go to work, but like zero-hours contractors they don't know where or when they are working today. They need some direction. Unluckily for them they don't have an app or agency to help and take a large percentage of their pay, but what they DO have is their old buddy CO_2.

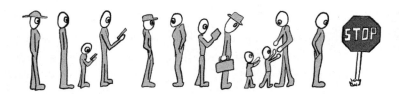

As the RBCs race around the body, driven by our ever-pumping heart, the bus driver looks out for any CO_2 molecules that may be flagging the RBCs down, and if there's any O_2 left on board then they make a neat and swift 1 for 1 swap. The CO_2 is what signals the release of O_2 to our cells. Without it the RBCs would continue to race around the body and return to our lungs still loaded with O_2.

The CO_2 actually breaks the bond that the RBCs have with the O_2, and once this is broken the O_2 is released into the cell that needs it to live, and the CO_2 molecule hitches aboard and is carried all the way round our body, back to our lungs and we exhale it out again.

After cell metabolism there is an excess of CO_2 on site. This is indeed a waste product and, if there is a considerable build-up or if it goes on for long enough, this can cause problems, as any build-up of waste products always does.

BUT - and this is the critical take-away point here - CO_2 is not bad in and of itself, and in fact it now performs a critical role by signalling to the RBCs where the oxygen is needed and then breaks the haemoglobin bond, freeing the oxygen to be able to do its job where it is most needed.

CO2 has become the foreman. CO2 has become the director of operations!

The urge to breathe is not low O2, but higher levels of CO2 in the blood. Specific CO2 chemoreceptors located in the body and brain, let us know when levels are too high and we exhale and inhale accordingly to bring the levels back down. This is mostly spoken about in the literature out there as 'balancing the PH in the body'. As excess CO2 is acidic, we need to bring the blood back to PH 7.35.

An interesting aside, is that one of these chemoreceptors is in our neck around where our clavicles are. This is why, when we are short on breath or holding our breath for a long time, we feel a tightness and uncomfortable constriction around this area.

CO2 isn't just something toxic that needs expelling from our body as fast as possible, it acts as a marker as to where we need O2 delivering. As cells work harder, and metabolism increases (let's think of a muscle cell during exercise), then more CO2 is released. This signals to passing RBC's that more O2 is required on site and energy is delivered to where it is most required at that time.

CO2 Paradox
The vast body of research has been drawn together by investigative scientists like Patrick Mckeown, and they have uncovered a hidden secret that has further changed our understanding and appreciation of CO2 and the role it plays in our body. He (and other, most significantly James Nester and Brian McKenzie), have demonstrated that CO2 and our relationship with this molecule can actually boost our mental and physical performance, and bring us greater levels of health.

Apart from being something that we need to expel as quickly as possible from our bodies, current understanding has it that we can benefit from training our bodies to be more tolerant of higher CO2 levels. This in turn enables us to almost supercharge our physical and mental abilities, and can crush anxiety and performance reducing aspects caused by 'stress'.

We can train our bodies to accept and perform under higher levels of CO2 to reach new highs. But how is this possible?

With time and training we can gradually let the levels of CO2 build up in our body. *The Oxygen Advantage* includes all the necessary exercises to perform, and there's a network of qualified coaches / instructors worldwide (of which I am one) who can help you on a more personal level. By gradually and temporarily increasing our levels of CO2 in the body, we are nudging-up the ability of our body to tolerate CO2's presence without going into a stressed or anxious state.

When the chemoreceptors detect high or uncomfortable levels of CO2 in the body, this triggers a feeling of stress. However, how we interpret these bodily sensations also plays a major role in how severe the stress response will be. If we are able to withstand higher levels of CO2, then we simply won't interpret this as 'stress 'and we're therefore able to stop many of the negative feedback loops that would otherwise kick in at this point, and start that spiral out of our control into anxiety and even panic.

So, if we can reprogram or reset our interpretation of, or our tolerance to, CO2, then we can redefine what we find or feel as stressful. We put ourselves firmly back in control.

For our purposes, this means two essential things:
* We are able to tolerate higher levels of CO2 in the blood, so the stress 'alarm 'that goes off when CO2

levels get too high is less sensitive. Like the ideal smoke alarm in our kitchen, it knows the difference between a bit of burnt toast and a chip-pan or electrical fire.

- We are able to utilise this increase in CO_2 levels to signal to our RBCs that we need more O_2. This means we can get an increase of O_2 delivered to our cells and we can perform past our previous limits. We are now able to meet a higher demand for O_2, growing stronger and increasing our endurance.

Through the simple act of performing light and low breathing practices (see Chapter 12 and 'My Go-to Exercises' for more details) and specific breath-holding exercises we are able to increase our tolerance of CO_2, both increasing our performance and decreasing our general stress levels.

Athletes the world over are now harnessing this knowledge to incorporate breathwork into their training routines. The benefits include a clear mind, better cognition and faster decision-making under pressure as well as increased athletic ability, it terms of both for strength and endurance.

Pretty life-changing stuff and all just from a few breathing techniques!

Balance is Still Key

Despite these findings, and that some athletes and scientists claiming that this can make us superhuman - achieving more than we ever thought possible, and in shorter times, with a less harmful impact on the body, we should return to the old principle that balance is indeed key.

Being able to tolerate higher levels of CO_2 is a goal all of us can and should strive for. The benefits, from athletic prowess to a freer creative flow and better sleep, helps all of us, in all aspects of our lives. But this **doesn't** mean that we should strive for higher levels of CO_2 in our body *all* of the time.

It still remains true that for most of us, constant higher levels of CO2 in the body will result in damage, illness and a premature death. We shouldn't strive to maintain high levels of CO2 but likewise we shouldn't be scared of it. We can train our bodies to be more tolerant of higher levels and perform more effectively under those conditions.

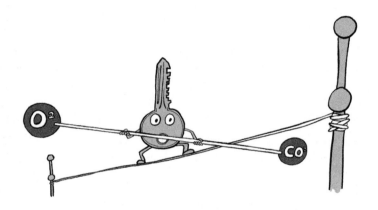

Carbon dioxide has been much maligned and misunderstood in the past but now our understanding has expanded and grown to put this to rights. CO2 is essential in healthy respiration. It helps us in *how* we breathe. Higher levels of CO2 in the blood are detected in the chemoreceptor sensors and this triggers our need to breathe. This can also be interpreted as stress in the body, and a continued state results in rising anxiety.

We can utilise temporarily high levels of CO2 to our advantage and we can also train ourselves to literally not get so stressed about the slightly rising levels, after all, this helps us increase our O2 delivery. But we do not want to make high levels of CO2 *on its own* our aim. Like all life on earth, and possibly further afield, we need to seek balance.

The even better news is that all these breathing exercises are readily available and with correct training we can see improvements very quickly.

There are more exercises at the end of the book but again, the one I always turn to is the aptly named 'Old Faithful'.

So next time we see those 'Wanted Dead or Alive 'posters up for CO_2 let's at least take some time to think about what context they're being used in. Now we know more of the 'back story', let's think about who's saying it and why, and maybe it's even time to peel that poster off the wall. We're not chasing the bounty but addressing the real problems and maybe becoming a breathwork hero in the process!

Chapter 10
Awareness

For me one of the most valuable aspects of breathwork and healthy everyday breathing, is the stillness and the connection it has brought to me, myself and my surroundings. Breathwork has been practised in many guises since we first became aware. Perhaps we became aware because we started practising forms of breathwork?

Every ancient religion incorporates and embraces breathwork in some form or another, whether it be through chanting, singing, meditation or direct breath-control exercises. Ancient yogis knew what the score was and modern science is only just catching-up with their teachings now.

The Gateway into our Body

The value of focusing on our breath and drawing our attention inwards, helps us find a level of calm and self knowledge that we only dreamed of previously. We find that we can now understand the subtle cues our body gives us, and we're able to not only listen to them but also instinctively know what needs to be done. This moves us from imbalance and pain or danger, and towards growth and homeostasis.

The 'Old Faithful 'exercise is my go-to and is an amalgamation of many practices out there. It is simple enough to be performed anywhere and under any conditions (except maybe not swimming for our life while being chased by a Great White with a newly discovered taste for human flesh - but here's hoping that scenario doesn't pop-up).

Breathing and breathwork is a gateway into our body, it enables us to follow physical cues deeper into ourselves, to listen to what's really going on. Our brains are amazing, but as our patterns are built on the years and decades of bad decisions, parental advice, blind luck and confirmation bias it's no wonder that the conclusions we might jump to could go a little askew.

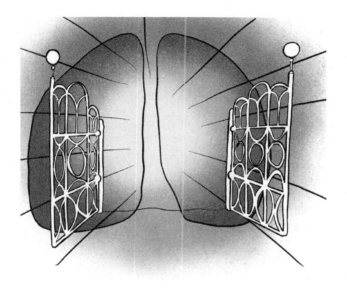

If your mind is anything like mine, it doesn't often have my best interests at heart. Rather, my internal dialogue certainly doesn't serve my best interests and if anything, holds me back. I'd never speak to a stranger as harshly as I speak to myself.

Focusing on my breath allows me to really feel what *is* and not what is imagined.

By going deeper in my practices I'm able to hear my internal dialogue, but with a detached and bemused air about it all. I'm able to see these strange conclusions, 'beliefs' and 'truths' carved in stone for the shams they are, and this has brought me a greater level of freedom in my life.

One Small Step and a Recap

By now you will be noticing more how you breathe in your daily life. Just by bringing our attention to something heightens our awareness of it. It sharpens the image and brings it into focus.

The same is true of our breath. Just buying this book, borrowing it or receiving it as a gift) started this process, and the more you have read the more aware you have probably become of your breath - perhaps becoming fascinated or borderline obsessed.

This is normal and good.

We are taught aspects of health at school and elsewhere, but our breath is almost always forgotten. So this hard remembering, this shoulder-shake back into reality, is a very beneficial thing and something to be celebrated.

Simply being more aware of our breath means we will breathe better.

This is one of the best kept secrets out there, so if you share just one thing share this. It can be done in any professional setting or even over your third pint. Once this seed is sown, only good things can blossom from it. Maybe the person you tell will sign up to a local breathwork class, watch a meditation on YouTube, shave their head and move to India - or better still, will rush out and buy a copy of this book!

Hallelujah!

We have looked at how we breath and how it affects us on a physiological and mental level. We have seen that over-breathing causes a stress response and we have explored why this is and what we can do about it. We have dived a little deeper and looked at why we breathe in the first place and hopefully connected some dots as to why then our breathing affects us so deeply. It is one of the cornerstones of our life.

We have put two and two together as to why, when we are short of breath it feels unpleasant and why our attention falters, drifts and flys clean out the window - oh look! Squirrels! We have also explored how ineffective breathing and stress makes us feel tired all the time - except of course when we need to go to sleep, then we just lie there with a racing mind unable to get to sleep!

We have identified the two buttons at our disposal: the Big Red Button in our chest to activate our sympathetic nervous system - our 'fight and flight 'and the big blue button in our belly - or rather, on our diaphragm which stimulates the parasympathetic nervous system, calming things down and giving us the space to 'rest and digest'.

These things were, or seemed, out of our control until very recently. It's part of the reason it's called the autonomic nervous system - and we were expected to be silent victims of our own cruel destiny. But now we know that we ARE in control. That we have access to these two buttons and a whole lot more besides.

The more aware of things we are, the more able we are to practise reversing or slowing any destructive processes within us, and the greater the benefits will be. The more often we can do this, the better and more self-serving (in a good way) our feedback loops become. We create new neural pathways and the more natural it becomes.

One day, when sitting at our computer, the pop-up calendar tells you that our taxes are due. Instead of hiding our computer in a dark drawer or throwing it out of the window, closing the blinds and turning the music up loud... we simply take a deep diaphragmatic breath without even realising it and casually start thinking about doing our taxes.

Extra Strings of the Awareness Bow

We recognise what's going on in our body. We start to connect external and internal triggers and the responses they generate. We start to understand the changes we can easily make to stay in control, and before we know it these things are happening naturally and without any overt or conscious effort.

We then start to be able to positively use our breathwork tools to start unpicking all those other issues that lie just beneath the surface. Giving ourselves the calm space we often lack, and allowing the blood-flow to open-up previously blocked or deliberately locked parts of our brain and memory, we are able to delve deep into our un/sub-conscious.

Some really 'magical 'things start to happen at this stage too. Because we are getting more adept at feeling into our bodies, and listening to the cues the internal systems are giving us, we start to become more body-aware in general.

We start actually listening to our body instead of trying to overpower it and beat it into submission. When we feel tired we start to take power-naps instead of forcing coffee down our throats. We start to feel unknown urges towards healthier food options and our taste starts improving too. It's almost as if our bodies *know* what we need and have been communicating to our deaf ears all along. A deep sense of relief and relaxation rushes in.

And this isn't surprising. Modern society is a deafening place. We are constantly bombarded with adverts telling us what we need, what we will enjoy and what we should be doing. Sugar, fat and salt hits reinforce this narrative and we sink into a blissful but chronically sick state of being.

When we listen to our bodies, when we start doing and eating what we need, we find this positive feedback loop just keeps growing stronger every day. With our increased tolerance to stress, and therefore uncomfortable feelings, we are able to notice the adverts and sugar-coated cravings for what they are, and slowly start saying goodbye to them.

This doesn't turn us into saintlike nutritionists but it does nudge us further in the right direction and again gives us positive reinforcements to the good decisions we are now taking. Our impulsive and destructive cravings are replaced by our true and wonderful gut feeling, driven by billions of bacteria whose life depends upon us!

All of this starts by bringing more awareness to our breath. Pretty cool really!

Chapter 11
Bringing it All Together

If you'd have told my younger old self that I would be happily breathing through my nose in my forties, I'd have thought you were smoking crack, unless you were Marty McFly trying to get *Back to the Future* - and then maybe I'd have listened to you.

Hindsight though is a wonderful thing, and I now realise that correct breathing practices, and why we should do them should absolutely be taught in primary school and then incorporated as normal practice as school progresses. Special sessions should be held during especially trying times, like when preparing for exams, and of course in sports classes too.

This book is by no means a comprehensive and complete look at the world of functional breathing and breathwork. Most of us don't even have enough time in our lives to read all of the literature out there, but I hope you've found it a useful and entertaining companion. This area of health and wellbeing is one that's certainly worth disappearing down the rabbit hole with. Just beware of the extreme videos out there with a million likes. Stick to the basics and you can't go wrong.

So as not to leave you in the lurch, and although I am actually a big fan of re-reading books, I'm also a fan of a nice recap. So here's a handy, if not a comprehensive review of everything we've covered so far.

Deep Breath (Efficient, but not over-breathing)

A deep breath is a full breath - or as full as you need. Deep signifies the furthest from the surface rather than all-out effort and hyperventilating.

With your breath starting at your diaphragm, breathe in through the nose at a nice controlled rate.

This will allow everything in the respiratory system to work as it has evolved to do.

Sleep and nose breathing

By breathing better during the day, and helping to manage stress levels, we will fall asleep more easily.

Then once in the land of nod, we'll be able to go into all the different stages of sleep due to peaceful nasal breathing (maybe with the use of mouth tape).

Our body is able to rest, repair, recover and recharge ready for the next day and whatever life throws at us.

Balancing Bodily Systems

As we take our nice deep and balanced breaths, this will bring equilibrium to the rest of our body's systems. We are able to digest and extract all the nutrients from our food, and feed our cells and natural growth through repair and renewal, as efficiently as possible.

Our hormonal and neurological systems will be working optimally and as such so will our heart and other aspects of our cardio-vascular system.

Fixing Sitting! Posture!

This is a chicken and egg situation but with good posture comes great breathing, and with great breathing comes unstoppable posture and core strength.

Sit well with an open posture and reap the benefits all day. Though don't forget to get up once in a while and shake it all off!

Stress!

High levels of stress affects the way we breathe, and conversely how we breathe affects how stressed we become. We can over-breathe and hyperventilate all day long, pushing ourselves into chronic stress or we can slow it down, breathing through our nose and belly and chill the hell out.

Press the Big Red Button or the Big Blue Button. The choice is yours, Nemo.

Bingeing and Burnout

With lower stress we are less likely to feel the need to binge on sugary and fatty foods, our need to find satisfaction through stimulants, drugs and alcohol can decrease as we find we have the coping mechanisms built within us.

We are less likely to race happily towards collapse, and as such can focus on wellbeing and longevity instead of sickness and recovery. But if we have taken the second route, we can soon navigate back to the first, after a little intervention.

Sports Performance and Recovery

Better oxygen flow will ensure greater energy during performance.

Switching fast chest breaths to deep diaphragmatic breaths will increase recovery in between rounds and after sports.

Deep sleep, due to better breathing, will enable faster muscle growth and repair after exhaustion, getting you back on the pitch again, faster.

Concentration, Focus (and athletic performance from strength to endurance)

With good breathing practices, our concentration is better and our focus is clearer and more sustainable.

Our athletic performance is better wherever we may be active, and our strength and endurance improves.

With faster recovery we feel almost unstoppable!

Increase Productivity and Feeling Happier!

Put simply, we are able to do more, are able to relax properly and just feel a damn sight better.

So here we go then, let's take a nice slow deep breath in through the nose into our diaphragm, feeling the belly grow slightly as we inhale. Our ribs start to move outwards and we feel an opening around our heart. A lightness starts to flood through the body and we smile to ourselves.

You're a breathing badass and you are unstoppable!

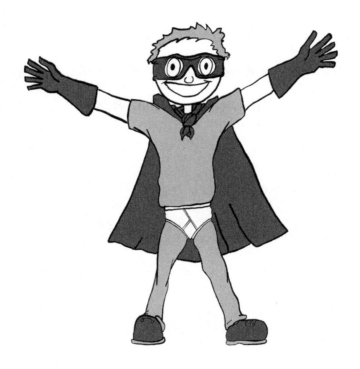

Congratulations!
YOU are a
Breathing Bad-Ass
and Super Hero!

Chapter 12
My Go-to Exercises

Here's a little reference of all my favourite breathing exercises. It was really tempting to write a comprehensive list but this would soon become a rather dry and perhaps disingenuous encyclopaedia of breathing techniques.

Everyone is different and everyone will breathe differently at different times in our lives, weeks and days. For example, for anyone menstruating or on HRT, progesterone can seriously affect the body's ability to uptake oxygen by around 20%. As we have also seen, stress, diet, and sleep all affect our breath, this is also one of the reasons I never time my breath-holds.

So instead I'll continue to preach what I practise and here is a small selection of exercises and techniques that I will use at least once a week. Find what works best for you, keep learning and discovering new techniques and make them your own. But, also let's not forget that the foundation techniques are the 'basic building blocks 'for a reason.

Breathe Light

This is a basic go-to which I practise multiple times a day. If you'd like to learn more you can read *The Oxygen Advantage* as this is a staple of Patrick McKeown's work.

Our aim here is to slowly decrease the amount we are breathing to gently build-up 'air hunger 'and carbon dioxide levels. This nudges our ability to tolerate higher levels of carbon dioxide.

- Start breathing normally, bringing our awareness within. Notice how the breath moves in and out of the body.

- See if you can feel your heart beating in your chest. This can take a long time, don't rush it or feel frustrated. Once you can feel your heartbeat, see if you can feel into the connection between breath and heartbeat.
- Notice how you are breathing and if you are breathing through the mouth, slowly switch to your nose.
- Bring your awareness to the tip of your nose. Feel the air flowing in and then relaxing and flowing out again.
- Slowly, every few breaths, start to breathe a little lighter, a little less than you feel you should be inhaling.
- You should be feeling gentle 'air hunger 'not a strong urge to breathe.
- If you need to gasp for air, rather than pick up where you left off, simply smile, and start the process again.

Walking Exercises
NOTE - if you are a jogger, try these first when walking but then incorporate them into your runs, starting at the beginning and then building-up to as far as you can go.

Nasal Breathing All the Way
- First and foremost, nasal breathing is the most important thing to remember.
- Our aims are to increase our ability to nose breathe, to open-up our airways and cardio-vascular system and bring balance into the body. We are also increasing our tolerance to carbon dioxide while also getting a cheeky little fitness workout.
- We match our pace to our breath and not the other way around.
- If we need to mouth breath then simply slow-down or stop and start the exercise again.
- It's fun! It's a journey. Don't beat yourself up if your 'fail', but notice when demand becomes too great and see if you

can *feel* into why that is. For example, is it a hill or the coffee you just had?

- If you are running, it is OK to employ the common 80:20 rule.

(Note: The 80:20 rule here means trying to do something for 80% of the time, rather than aiming for perfection - or 100% - all the time.)

Controlled Active Breath-holds

As well as conscious breathwork sessions a few times a week, I also practise breath-holding games every time I leave the house.

These can be done on your 'walks to the shop', while walking the dog or just when getting some fresh air and moving the body.

Note - these are NOT extreme breath-holds. Start small and build up. If you feel lightheaded you have pushed yourself too far so scale it back. Safety first!

- While walking, exhale normally and at a steady pace, count out your number of steps until you feel a need to inhale.
- Continue walking and breathing normally for a minute (nasally if you can of course)
- Repeat the exercise but see how many more steps you can take without increasing the need to breathe too much.
- Rest and repeat.
- Try again a few more times, but now try to comfortably push a little further.
- Finish on a few nice short breath-holds and nasal breathing.
- If you go uphill one way and down the other (as I do to my 'corner shop') notice the difference between the two!

NOTE: You should never push these too hard, as passing out while standing-up is dangerous! Also, they should be fun. Think of them as games or warm-ups for later exercise.

Old Faithful

This is my go-to breathwork exercise and it fits pretty much any occasion and situation.

- Close your eyes and give yourself permission to stop, whether it is lying down or just stepping away from the computer or the office.

- Stopping is the most important first step.

- Now feel into your breath, notice how you are breathing, you aren't trying to change how you're breathing, you aren't judging how you're breathing, we are just noticing it.

- Nice.
  Now slowly, slowly, start to inhale just using your diaphragm.

- Just breathe in and out as your body sees fit, but just use your diaphragm, feel your belly expand and contract with each breath.

- Smile into your breath and let yourself go.

- Set an alarm for three to five minutes if pressed for time, or just keep going if you're able to.

Longer Exhales

This one is so simple it's almost criminal it's not taught to children.

- To down-regulate or to balance out, overactive nervous systems, simply exhale for a longer count than your inhale.

- If you can incorporate a natural pause after the inhale - even better.
  That's it and it works great!

(Free-Diving) Overload

This will force the excess oxygen into our blood. It is great as an energising pick-me-up mid morning or afternoon, or whenever the mood takes me.

(We need to be *really* careful not to hyperventilate before going in or under water. I was taught this method to fully pack the lungs on one breath before diving down.)

- We start with minute of light and relaxation breathing, slowing the heart and breath.
- Then we take one deep breath in, almost swallow it deep down and then fill it up with another breath on-top to 'double-load'.

Wim Hof Breathing

This is a powerful breathing technique that I do first thing in the morning every other day or more often depending on how I am feeling. Put safety FIRST - lie or sit down and check out the health contraindications first.

I'd recommend learning this properly from a professional Instructor and then tailor it best to your own physiology. With permission, from the WHM Official Website: www.wimhofmethod.com

1 - Assume a meditation posture: sitting, lying down - whichever is most comfortable for you. Make sure you can expand your lungs freely without feeling any constriction.

2 - 30-40 Deep Breaths
Close your eyes and try to clear your mind. Be conscious of your breath, and try to fully connect with it. Inhale deeply through the nose or mouth, and exhale unforced through the mouth. Fully inhale through the belly, then chest and then let go

unforced. Repeat 30 to 40 times in short, powerful bursts. You may experience light-headedness, and tingling sensations in your fingers and feet. These side effects are completely harmless though can be disorientating to the uninitiated.

3 - The Hold
After the last exhalation, inhale one final time, as deeply as you can. Then let they air out and stop breathing. Hold until you feel the urge to breathe again.

4 - Recovery Breath
When you feel the urge to breathe again, draw one big breath to fill your lungs. Feel your belly and chest expanding. When you are at full capacity, hold the breath for around 15 seconds, then let go. That completes round number one. This cycle is repeated 3-4 times without interval. After having completed the breathing exercise, take your time to bask in the bliss. This calm state is highly conducive to meditation - don't hesitate to combine the two.

Box Breathing
Similar to my 'Old Faithful', box breathing is an exercise which I may employ a few times a day to bring balance, clarity and focus.
This was supposedly developed by the Navy SEALs to stay sharp, and get ready for a tactical operation, but it's just as effective and applicable if you're getting ready for a meeting or after the school run.

It's simple and effective and should be one of your go-to breathwork tools. For the drummers out there, it's basically the 'Standard 8th Note Groove' for breathwork.
- Breathe in for a count of four.
- Hold for a count of four.
- Exhale for a count of four.
- Hold for a count of four.

- Repeat for a few minutes or until you feel balanced and focussed.

NOTE: You can alter the count to twos, threes, fives or sixes, whichever works best for you as long as they are consistent and each 'side of the square 'is the same length.

Sometimes I like to combine Box Breathing with walking and nasal breathing.

The Nodder

This technique is great for unblocking our nose. It works by confusing our body into thinking we can't breathe, and letting the NO2 build up. So that when we inhale, an overload of nitric acid does its magic, and everything opens up naturally.

- Inhale and exhale normally.
- Pinch your nose and breathe very gently into the cavity around your nose (like you do when trying to acclimatise on an aeroplane).
- As you gently exhale into this space, nod very deliberately - but not head-banging.
- Nod 5 - 20 times, or whenever you feel a need to breathe again.
- Let go of your nose and slowly inhale through it.

Breath 'normally 'for about 30 seconds and then
Repeat five times

My Daily Breathwork Schedule and Getting Started!

I try to keep everything as simple as possible. Through years of practice I can often feel what kind of practice my body needs before I begin.

However, simply following the three-step process outlined in 'Old Faithful' is always a great place to start, and helps us focus on the task of breathing itself, and how we feel in our bodies, at that time.

It's always too easy to skip a practice like breathwork or think 'I'll do it later'. On those days when I'm yawning by 10.30 am I often gently berate myself as, almost without fail, it will because I had skipped my morning breathwork and/or cold shower. Whatever excuse we come up with, dedicating just a few minute first thing in the morning will bring benefits throughout the day.

After a few minutes of listening to my body, letting my mind be still, and feeling into my new day, I will either practise Breathing Light or I will go straight into a self-guided version of the WHM (Copyright) Breathing. Most people find this too difficult, especially at first so there are plenty of excellent free YouTube videos and there is a paid-for WHM App.

I then stretch, shake it out, and sometimes exercise, then I have a warm then cold shower and it is on with the day!

Mid-morning and mid-afternoon, I like to practise a balancing breath - Breathing Light, Box Breathing or my Old Faithful, which is always a great one for the first few months of getting started. Remember, you are in for the long haul and not just a sprint.

If I am lucky, in the evening I will attend a guided breathwork class or self-guide myself at home, although most evening I work guiding others so this is a luxury. Some evenings, I just need to crumple on the sofa...

Before bed I again focus on balancing out my breath again, often bringing my heart rate back down again, and then as I am reading I'll Breathe Light until I feel my eyes start to close.

Then it's time to lay my book down, turn off the light and smile to myself before drifting into a multi-coloured night of dreams.

My biggest three tips would be:

- Start slow.
- Do what works best for *you*. Take advice and guidance from others, but only you know what works for you - and becoming able to *really* listen to your body's needs is one of the greatest gifts of all.
- Lastly: have fun! Play, develop new patterns and sequences. If you enjoy it, you will continue long after this book has been lent to a friend.

Bibliography and Further Reading

Brulé, Dan 'Just Breathe: *Mastering Breathwork*' (2017), New York, First Enliven Books / Atria

Burhenne, Dr. Mark (DDS) 'The 8-Hour Sleep Paradox: *How We Are Sleeping Our Way To Fatigue, Disease & Unhappiness* (2015) Sunnyvale, Independently Published

Carney, Scott 'What Doesn't Kill Us: *How freezing water, extreme altitude, and environmental conditioning will renew our lost evolutionary strength* (2017), Melbourne/London: Scribe

Carney, Scott 'The Wedge: *Evolution, Consciousness, Stress and the Key to Human Resilience*' (2020), Denver: Foxtopus Ink

Case, R.M. & Waterhouse 'Human Physiology: *Age, Stress and the Environment*' (1997), Oxford, Oxford Science Publications

Clear, James 'Atomic Habits: *An Easy and Proven Way to Build habits & Break Bad Ones* (2018), London, Random House

Drake, Richard, L (PHD), Vogl, Wayne A (PHD) & Mitchell, Adam W.M. (MB, BS, FRCS, FRCR)' Gray's Anatomy for Students: *4th Edition* '(2019), Amsterdam, Elsevier

Evans, Emily, 'Anatomy In Black', 2016 Chichester, Lotus Publishing

Hof, Wim 'The Wim Hof Method: *Activate Your Potential, Transcend Your Limits* (2020), London, Penguin / Random House

Limmer, Daniel, O'Keefe, Michael F & Dickenson, Edward T (M.D., FACEP) 'Emergency Care: *10th Edition*' (2005), New Jersey, Pearson Education Inc.

Mader, Sylvia S. et al 'Understanding Human Anatomy and Physiology: *Fifth Edition*' (2005), New York, McGraw-Hill

McGuire, Mike 'Freediving Manual: *How to Freedive 100 feet on a Single Breath (Freediving in Black and White)*' (2017), Independently Published

McKeown, Patrick 'The Oxygen Advantage: *The SImple Scientifically Proven Breathing Technique that will Revolutionise Your Health and Fitness* (2015), London: Piatkus

McKeown, Patrick 'The Breathing Cure: *Exercises to Develop New Breathing Habits for a Healthier and Longer Life*' (2021), Ireland, OxyAt Books

Nester, James 'Breath: *The New Science of a Lost Art*' (2020), London, Penguin / Random House

Rama (Swami), Ballentine, R (MD) & Hymes, A (MD) 'Science of Breath: *A Practical Guide* (1979), Honeysdale, Himalayan Institute

Starrett, Dr, Kelly with Cordoza, Glen 'Becoming a Supple Leopard: *The Ultimate Guide to Resolving Pain, Preventing Injury, and Optimizing Athletic Performance*' (2013), Las Vegas, Victory Belt Publishing Inc.

Tolle, Eckhart 'Practising The Power Of Now: *A Guide to Spiritual Enlightenment*' (2002) London, Yellow Kite Books

Vranich, Dr. Belisa and Sabin, Brian 'Breathing for Warriors: *Master Your Breath to Unlock More Strength, Greater Endurance, Sharper Precision, Faster Recovery, and an Unshakable Inner Game '*(2020), New York, St. Martins Publishing Group

Further Scientific Papers Reference

Chapter 4

The Nose

Svensson, S. Olin A.C. & Hellgren (2006) **Increased net water loss by oral compared to nasal expiration in healthy subjects,** Rhinology, 44, pp 74-77
https://www.rhinologyjournal.com/Rhinology_issues/554.pdf

Chapter 7

Stress and out Immune System

Liu, Yun-Zi, Wang, Yun-Xia & Jiang, Chun-Lei (2017) **Inflammation: The Common Pathway of Stress-Related Diseases,** Frontiers in Human Neuroscience

https://www.ncbi.nlm.nih.gov/pmc/articles/PMC5476783/

Schipani, D. (2023) **Here's How Stress and Inflammation Are Linked,** Everyday Health

Kox, M et al (2014) **Voluntary activation of the sympathetic nervous system and attenuation of the innate immune response in humans,** PNAS

https://www.wimhofmethod.com/cache/uploads/kcfinder/files/PNAS.pdf

Krueger, J. M. (2009) **The Role of Cytokines in Sleep Regulation,** PubMed Central

https://www.ncbi.nlm.nih.gov/pmc/articles/PMC2692603/

Besedovsky, L., Lange, T. & and Born, J. (2011) **Sleep and immune function,** PubMed Central

https://www.ncbi.nlm.nih.gov/pmc/articles/PMC3256323/

Printed in Great Britain
by Amazon